BODYWEIGHT
MUSCLE

By Anthony Arvanitakis

*A Science-Based Approach To Gaining
Mass Without Lifting Weights*

Dedicated to all the Bodyweight-Muscle supporters. Thank you for believing in me and keeping me motivated to motivate you.

Keep on training!

CONTENTS

This book is the result of years of research and self-experimentation.

It's the book I would like to have had when I first began my journey into bodyweight training. Having made a lot of personal mistakes, having followed a lot of bad advice, and having neglected a lot of important principles, I know that having this book back then would have saved me a lot of time and wasted effort.

Nowadays, I believe that I have found all the pieces of the puzzle that one needs to build an impressive physique and get in great shape through bodyweight exercise. And even though I can't go back in time to avoid my mistakes, I can help those of you who are either getting started on your journey or those that have been training for some time without getting the results that you should be getting and deserve...

INTRODUCTION

D uring this book, I refer to bodyweight training also by using the term calisthenics. There is a bit of confusion and a vagueness when it comes to this term, since people use it in different ways. Following is my personal definition of calisthenics and what I mean by using it.

Let's start with the origin of calisthenics. Calisthenics comes from the ancient Greek words kalos (κάλλος) and sthenos (σθένος). Kalos means beauty, which refers to the pleasure given by the sight of a very aesthetic human body. Sthenos is a form of mental strength that combines courage, braveness and determination. As a Greek person, and because I like how the word Calisthenics relates etymologically to what bodyweight training means for me, I use both words synonymously. Calisthenics/Bodyweight training is the art of using your own bodyweight to develop your physical fitness and sculpt your physique. Proper calisthenics training should make you stronger and improve your physique, but also at the same time promote general health.

Calisthenics shouldn't be confused with Urban Calisthenics (UC) – aka street workouts. These include more advanced and gymnastic-oriented skills, such as muscle ups, bars spins, levers, etc. Although UC are impressive and fun to practice, they are not ideal for most people past their thirties, or those prone to injury in general. Acute and long-term overuse-related injuries are common in UC. This is mostly caused by highly explosive movements or exercises that require extreme stabilization which multiply the tension your joints must absorb.

Take the front-lever, for example. This is a static hold normally performed on a pull-up bar from an inverted hang, where the body is completely horizontal and straight (with the front of the body facing upwards). No matter how progressive and strategic you are with your training approach to this skill, if you have sensitive elbows you will eventually start experiencing problems. Back in 2014 I was experimenting with some UC training and one of the skills I was working on was the front-lever. Although I did manage to achieve this skill after practicing for a couple of months, it also caused me elbow-pain which only subsided when I laid off this practice. I also tried other UC exercises, but I found that most of them came with a cost in the long run. No matter how careful you are, unless you have a background of a gymnast growing up, these exercises have a high risk of injury for most people.

After training and hanging out with a lot of talented, impressive urban calisthenic athletes in The Netherlands where I lived for seven years, I discovered that many of them suffered with issues even at young ages below twenty-five. Elbow and shoulder inflammation related problems were the most common thing. Here's the thing with UC: they might look super cool and fun when you stumble upon them on Youtube, but what you have to realize is that for every cool urban athlete we see doing impressive moves, there are a lot of other people that tried doing the same things and eventually got injured. Plus, notice how most of these guys and gals are in their early 20's. Rarely do you see people in their 40's or 50's doing the same thing. Sure, there are exceptions but as the saying goes "exceptions just prove the rule".

Don't get me wrong, I'm not saying I'm against UC. I think it's an awesome sport, but like most sports – it's not for everyone. Here's my advice if you want to add some more skill-oriented UC-related exercises to your routine. Find exercises that are joint-friendly and that don't stress parts of your body that might be already sensitive and prone to injury. For example, I like practicing handstands. These can stress the wrists a bit, but if you keep your wrists healthy with mobility and targeted conditioning exercises (such as wrist push-ups), it can be an fun implementation to most people's workout plan.

CALISTHENICS: A LONG-TERM RECIPE TO FITNESS, HEALTH AND LONGEVITY

The key thing to remember here is that if you're constantly getting hurt from your training – you're not training properly. Exercise should prevent injuries – not cause them. A proper calisthenics program should strengthen your muscles and connective tissues in a balanced way. It should keep your joints healthy and improve mobility. Strength and joint/connective tissue health are essential for long-term fitness. Sarcopenia (muscle-loss that occurs as you grow old) and lack of relative strength (how strong you are in relation to your bodyweight) are two of the most important reasons our bodies grow old.

There are studies showing a high correlation between bodyweight mobility and mortality. For example, a professor at the South Paul university found that there is a large correlation between your ability to get up off the floor and mortality. In his study, the more limbs/points of dependence one needed to get off the floor, the higher the correlation was with dying from all causes. When we think of age, we only think of it in a chronological way. But this is just one way we age and only one criterion to measure it. Not every sixty-year-old person has the same physical age for example. There are people in great physical condition at age sixty, and vice versa. Physical fitness reflects in our general age and health. A person that is in great shape will (most of the time) have better bloodwork results, a greater potential for longevity plus improved mental health compared to an immobile person.

Muscle mass ratio, mobility, relative strength... these are things that I think make a better biomarker for estimating how old your body is instead of just counting how many candles are on your birthday-cake. Lastly, being able to handle your own bodyweight with grace deep into old age is something important for all of us. It keeps us independent and able to enjoy life to it's outmost potential. And what better way to develop these characteristics than Bodyweight Exercise. A proper calisthenics routine works on natural movements that build functional muscle, while improving overall athleticism. It has the potential to be a long-term recipe for staying fit, healthy and maintaining a young body through time...

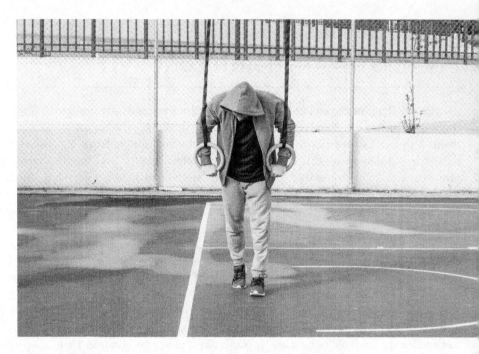

"Proper Bodyweight-training should prevent injuries – not cause them".

~ Bodyweight Muscle

CAN YOU REALLY BUILD MUSCLE ONLY WITH BODYWEIGHT TRAINING?

It is often debated whether bodyweight training is as effective as weight-lifting for developing a strong, muscular and aesthetic physique. One argument is that your own bodyweight does not provide enough resistance for optimal hypertrophy (muscle-growth). This is a reasonable concern, especially for lighter folks. Here's the thing though... even if you don't weigh that much, recent research has shown that even using as little as 30% of the maximum weight you can lift is enough for building muscle effectively (more on this later on).

Another argument is that heavier folks are not able to perform a lot of bodyweight exercises in the beginning. This can be solved by finding easier regressions of exercises that you *can* do. Instead of normal pull-ups, for example, you can do assisted pull-ups. Or, instead of normal push-ups, you can do incline push-ups. As long as you focus on improving gradually every week, you're on the right path. Plus, people that start with a heavy body-weight and gradually lose excessive fat, end up having impressive relative-strength! It's like training with a weighted vest. As you remove layers of that vest (as you lose fat) you are gradually managing to add more reps and perform harder variations.

The third most common argument is that progressive overload is not possible, so you eventually hit a ceiling. "Wait... what is Progressive Overload (PO)?" For those who don't know, PO is the gradual increase of stress placed upon the body during strength related training. The PO principle states that you have to continuously increase the demands on your neuromuscular system in order to continue to make gains in muscle-size. Although adding weight is one way to achieve progressive overload, it's not the only one. There are actually a lot of them! For example:
- Manipulating training volume (i.e. how many sets you do per week)
- Focusing on perfect technical execution of each exercise
- Using harder variations of your exercises
- Using specialized training techniques (i.e. supersets and circuits)

We'll talk about all these later in the book, but for now I want to talk a bit about technical execution, and how using proper form can make a huge difference both for health and hypertrophy reasons.

It's always tempting to try do more before your technique is perfect. Either that means adding more weight if you're training in a gym or doing more reps if you're training bodyweight. The thing is that in order to effectively build muscle you need to work on specific rep ranges. Increasing reps with bad form is easy, and a typical mistake bodyweight-trainees make. Working on refining your technique throughout every workout and concentrating on muscle contraction (aka Mind-to-Muscle awareness) is crucial for building bodyweight muscle successfully. Even the most basic bodyweight exercises become very challenging if you work on them in this way.

Take for example my trainee Chris. Chris was a Taekwondo national champion as a teenager. On our first workout, among other exercises, I had him do some push-ups. Although Chris has done a ton of push-ups back in his training days, that day was the first time that he felt a pump in his chest muscles. And that was just after his first set! All I did was give him some basic technical guidelines:

a) keep your elbows close to your ribcage and the chest open (shoulder back and down) while performing the exercise
b) lean a bit forward and try to place a bit more weight on your arms, instead of leaning too much on your toes
c) go all the way down slowly, until your nose touches the floor
d) pause for half a second at the bottom position and push yourself up in a controlled way

Give these a try if you haven't done push-ups this way before. Yes, try them right now if possible! Don't worry, I'll be still here when you come back.

Ok, so how was that? I bet you changed your opinion about push-ups being an easy basic exercise, right?

Working on refining your form with every workout, and not adding more reps before your form feels close to perfect makes a big difference. Still, it's not easy. It is something that requires discipline, patience and setting aside your ego. The great thing with calisthenics is that in a way they force you to develop these virtues since you are limited in terms of external equipment. Tony Robins says that success is not about resources... but about resourcefulness. I like that quote. You see, the only barbell you have with bodyweight training is your own body. This means that you have to master every other training parameter to get the most out of it.

Simplicity and mastery of the basics is not only key in fitness – it's the secret to most things. People from Bruce Lee to Leonardo Da Vinci have stated this in one way or another. I find that this is a mindset that has great value in life, and bodyweight exercise is a great tool to sharpen it.

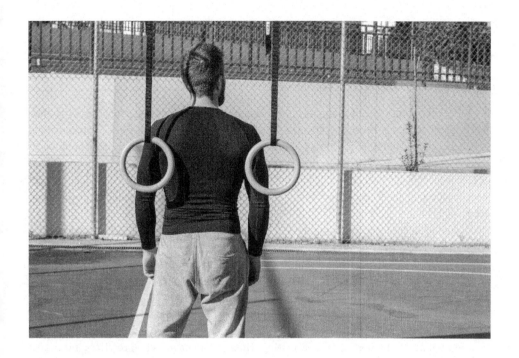

"Simplicity is the ultimate sophistication"

~ *Leonardo Da Vinci*

THE 4 BIGGEST BODYWEIGHT-TRAINING MISTAKES THAT ARE HOLDING YOU BACK

A lot of people contact me for help when they are lacking progress with their bodyweight workout routines. After years of answering these questions, I've narrowed down the main problems down to four categories. I decided to structure this book based on these:

1. Failing at the basics (not using proper rep-ranges, training volume, technique, etc.)
2. Nutrition (not getting enough protein, not eating enough or eating too much, etc.)
3. Not choosing the right exercises nor executing them the right way (i.e. using proper tempo, range of motion, focusing on muscle contraction, etc.)
4. Lack of programming (not having a well-thought out and long-term plan)

In Part 1 of the book you'll learn the essential Principles of building bodyweight muscle. Having a basic understanding of how your muscles grow and how rep-ranges, training volume (sets per week) and resting-time all affect muscle-growth is important. It will give you the proper foundation to start from.

A lot of your training can be also wasted if you don't fuel your body appropriately. This is why in Part 2 we'll discuss nutrition for building muscle and sculpting an impressive physique with bodyweight exercise. There are plenty of misconceptions in dieting that create confusion and often sabotage our goals. A lot of us (myself included in the past) tend to obsess over details and neglect very important basic nutritional principles that deliver most results in the long run. For most of us, when these basics are in order, ninety percent of our dietary issues are solved. This is enough for our body to start gradually taking the shape we want and keep us motivated to create a sustainable diet.

In Part 3 we'll talk about exercise selection and proper execution. Remember my friend Chris and the push-up example from before? There are a lot of bodyweight exercises to choose from, but only a few of them are worth your time and effort for building muscle and an impressive physique. Also, it's not just about choosing the right exercises – it's about performing them the right way.

In Part 4 I'll show you how to structure a long-term plan for maximizing muscle growth through the timespan of a year. There is also a ready-made plan for you to follow or use as a base-model upon which you can design your own plan. As the quote goes – *if you fail to plan, you are planning to fail*. You can only make so much progress by doing the same thing week after week.

BUILDING AN AESTHETIC BODYWEIGHT PHYSIQUE...

One of the reasons we all train is simply because we want to look in the mirror and like what we see. Sure, there are other reasons that we'll talk about later on (health, mood, etc.). Visual appeal though is always one of them – no matter how young or old you are. This is not a bad thing, especially when the by-product is living an overall healthier life. Now, before we talk about building bodyweight muscle and before you start setting goals, I consider it important that you start with a healthy mindset and reasonable expectations. After that, if you're methodical and follow the advice in this book, building a bodyweight physique that is both muscular and aesthetic will be a matter of time.

I think that most of us reading this book are not after the bodybuilding-contest type of physique. For those who are into that body, keep in mind that unless you have excellent genetics (google Arnold Schwarzenegger pictures from when he was a teenager), unless you're willing to risk your health with anabolic steroids and unless you don't care about having a healthy social life – it is very unlikely that you'll achieve this kind of physique. Plus, going after extremes is never a balanced approach... Look at muscle-dysmorphia (MD) for example. This is a common disorder in bodybuilding. In MD, the delusional or exaggerated belief is that one's own body is too small, too skinny, insufficiently muscular, or insufficiently lean; although in most cases, the individual's build is normal or even exceptionally large and muscular already. Eventually this can lead to abuse of illegal substances (i.e. steroids) and overtraining, to the extent that exercise takes more from your life instead of adding.

Here's my advice on how to set physique goals if you're just getting started:

1. Make sure that your goals are healthy (mentally and physically), and that exercise becomes part of your lifestyle but not your whole life.

2. Aim for a body that is "believably muscular" not that of a Hollywood actor with extreme genetics such as Dwayne Johnson. Think of the *"Goldilocks' principle"* here – not too big, not too small but just right for you.

3. We all have different body-types so respect the fact that not everyone can look like Bruce Lee, just like not everyone can look like Arnold Schwarzenegger. Some of us are meant to be slimmer and leaner. Others, with naturally bigger frames and bone structures, are meant to be more muscular and bulkier. And of course, there are countless of variations in between.

Learn to embrace what makes you happy. I'm not saying that you should settle for mediocre results. There's no doubt that you can change your body to a great extent. Just take things one step at time. If you have no abs at all, get started with aiming for a four-pack instead of a six-pack. Later, once you've trained in an organized fashion for at least a 6-7 months, you can reassess your goals and decide if you want to set up other more extreme ones.

Maybe you're happy with a four-pack and six extra pounds of muscle on your body. Maybe aiming for a six-pack and another four pounds of muscle will just make your life miserable. Or maybe you're so excited with your transformation that you want to keep pushing it. This is a choice that differs for everyone. What's more important is to find a balance and see what makes your life more functional and yourself happier. Overall, make sure that your fitness routine adds more quality to your life than it subtracts from it.

Now that we've covered all that, let's see how calisthenics can change your body. Here are the characteristics of someone with an aesthetic bodyweight physique:

- Relatively slim waist
- A healthy, low body-fat percentage
- Visible abs
- Round shoulders
- V-shaped defined back
- Visible muscular chest
- A pair of muscular and vascular arms
- Nicely shaped muscular legs

PART 1:
THE SCIENCE BEHIND
BUILDING MUSCLE WITH
CALISTHENICS

While writing this introductory part of the book I'm sitting in the train, on my way back home from a Sports & Performance Summit that took place in Amsterdam of the Netherlands. My mind wanders off a bit as I look outside the window at the typical Dutch scenery of green fields and cows. The past three days I had the honor of listening to world renowned authorities and researchers on muscle-hypertrophy, strength training and athletic nutrition. When I first started writing this book, I wasn't sure of how much science-oriented theory to put in it. But this summit reminded me of the importance of understanding basic scientific principles whenever you're serious about a goal in life.

Getting started...
Creating a proper workout plan is both complicated and simple. Complicated, because there are a lot of factors that come into play. "Are you training frequently enough?" "Are you resting too much or too little?" "Are you focusing on the right number of reps?" "Are you doing enough sets?" "Are you doing the right exercises?" It's normal to feel confused when it comes to these matters since there's such a large amount of conflicting information out there. Then again, creating a proper workout plan is also simple, because once you have the right answers to all these questions, it's just a matter of getting organized and putting a few things down on paper.

Another common motivational picture I see around social media says that all you need to do to build muscle is "Train, Eat, Rest, Repeat." Sure, in a way, if you oversimplify things, it does all boils down to that. But, that's also not the most helpful information when you're a newbie just past your beginner-gains period or if you're a hard-gainer (*someone who struggles a bit more than average to gain weight and muscle mass*). It's not even helpful for more advanced trainees since advanced plateaus are even more difficult to break.

Einstein said that "everything should be made as simple as possible but no simpler". Therefore, yes you have to train, but... are you training properly? Yes, you have to eat, but how much and what? Resting is required as well, but it should be optimized. Repeat sure, but at what frequency? Based on all this, I'd correct the previous quote to "Train properly, eat according to your needs and repeat in an ideal frequency that allows you to get in enough training volume while recovering optimally on a weekly basis." It's not as catchy a quote as it was previously, but you get my point! I'm all about simplicity when it comes to training, yet there are some things that must be properly structured. Even as an advanced trainee, maybe you can train a bit more instinctively, but for optimal progress... you simply cannot train randomly! Keeping track of your workouts, cycling hard training-periods with maintenance-periods, adjusting exercises, etc.... are all things you need to learn to do.

In Part 1, we'll cover basic hypertrophy principles. This will help you understand why you're doing what you're doing later on, and it will give you trust in the process and guidelines provided to you. It will also help you understand why some common advice and things you might have considered as standard fitness advice, is actually bad advice that don't make any sense whatsoever. There are a lot of fitness myths that have been perpetuated over the last few decades. This is why it's important to keep an open mind in case you read things that challenge some of your core beliefs.

Although I'll try to keep everything as simple as possible (but no simpler) and I will focus on the juicy stuff (I'll avoid using too much scientific theory and vocabulary)... keep in mind that you still might have to learn a few new exercise-science related terms.

THE SCIENCE BEHIND WHAT MAKES YOUR MUSCLES GROW

Muscles grow by repairing small micro-tears that occur on a cellular level during strength-training related exercise. When these tears occur, blood flow to the area increases in order to bring with it the necessary components for repair. When this process is over, the muscle becomes stronger and larger than before.

This rebuilding of the muscle is called Muscle Protein Synthesis (MPS). Whenever the rate of MPS is greater than the rate of muscle protein breakdown in your body, hypertrophy is the end result. As you might already know, most of this adaption does not happen while you train but while you rest.

A common misconception is that strength-training creates new muscle cells. What actually happens is that individual muscle cells increase in size. These bigger and stronger muscle cells are what give you a more aesthetically pleasing appearance. Underlying all progression of natural muscle growth is the ability to continually put more stress on the muscles. Based on the latest research, we know that there are three important mechanisms behind muscle-growth: a) Mechanical tension, b) Metabolic stress and c) Muscle damage.

Mechanical tension: When lifting weight, either that's your own bodyweight or an external weight (such as a dumbbell) your muscles are under tension which is called mechanical tension.

Metabolic stress: In simple words, metabolic stress is what causes that burning feeling you usually experience during mid- and high-rep training. Especially when you train close to momentary muscle failure and end up out of breath. The reason you feel that burning feeling is because you're depleting your muscles of oxygen. Also, that feeling when your muscles swell up after high-rep sets (aka the pump)? That's another thing related to metabolic stress. The mechanisms by which metabolic stress causes hypertrophy are still not entirely clear. The most established theory says that by promoting fatigue of slow-twitch fibers it forces activation the fast-twitch fibers.

Muscle damage: Exercise damage (or if you want to be more precise, exercise-induced-muscle-damage) is experienced as soreness during the first twenty-four to seventy-two (max) hours after a workout. This happens mostly when we first get started with a workout routine and haven't trained for a while. It can also happen when we switch things in our workout routine (like adding a new exercise). How significant is muscle-damage for hypertrophy? We still don't know... But don't worry, you don't have to feel sore all the time in order to build muscle since mechanical tension and metabolic stress are a lot more important. Some evidence also seems to show that too much soreness can be counterproductive and can even interfere with muscle-growth.

HOW HARD SHOULD YOU TRAIN?

Now that we've looked at the basic prerequisites for building muscle from a scientific perspective, let's also examine muscle-growth from a more empirical viewpoint. Despite some differences, if you study most people that are famous for their physiques, they all seem to agree on the following criteria when it comes to building an aesthetic body:

   a) Make training part of your lifestyle.
   b) Train focused (mute those social media!).
   c) Be methodical and keep track of your progress.
   d) Train hard and keep challenging yourself over time

We'll talk about points 1,2 and 3 later on in the book but right now I want to focus on the fourth point – Training hard. I think that this is one of the most important factors for muscle-growth and progress, yet it is also the one least talked about. Maybe one reason is that the amount you exert yourself is not something that is tangible such as sets, reps and resting periods, that are easily quantified through numbers.

It's a fact that you have to be producing enough intensity from each set and workout in order to disrupt your body's homeostasis (*maintenance of a stable condition in our body – aka an equilibrium*) if you want to trigger hypertrophy. Whether we like it or not, training hard enough is undoubtedly what has the greatest impact on our results. You won't build muscle if your training isn't challenging your muscles enough, not matter how frequent and how long you work out. I'd like to tell you that I have some amazing training secret to share with. One that allows you to by-pass the fact that you have to push yourself, but I don't.

So, how hard should you be training? Training hard means pushing yourself enough that you stimulate optimal muscle growth, but not too much that you end up injured or burned out halfway through your workout. You want to get close to or even reach failure after certain reps and sets of your workout. More on this in the next paragraph. Just keep in mind that you also want to avoid extremes though such as training till failure on every set (as some proponents of the "High Intensity Training Camp" advise). Unless you have out of the norm recovery abilities (or use steroids which I don't recommend), overdoing it this way is simply counterproductive.

MOMENTARY MUSCLE FAILURE (MMF)

I mentioned the importance of training close to or reaching failure in the previous paragraph. To be more specific, I was talking about Momentary Muscle Failure (MMF). This is the point you reach at the end of a set, after which you cannot perform another repetition with good form. It's important to be aware of this threshold. Once you feel things such as your body doing jerky moves or using momentum to get the next rep – you've reached that point.

Let's say you're doing pull-ups... For most of us, form in this exercise starts breaking down once we start extending our jaw to reach the bar. After that we usually start kicking with our feet and jerking our pelvis back and forth to swing ourselves up to the bar through momentum. When you feel you're beginning to extend your head to reach the bar, try to keep your head straight and see if you can get one or two more reps with no cheating at all. Focus as much as possible on smooth movement, clean form and muscle contraction during those last reps. Once you can't lift yourself anymore stop.

Another sign that our form is breaking down is muscle tension in the wrong places. Rounding and tensing your shoulders during push-ups or dips is a good example.

I don't recommend reaching MMF in every single set, but rather finding the right number of repetitions that result in reaching MMF during the last set of each exercise. Here's what I mean: let's say part of your training today has you doing four sets of dips. You don't want to go so hard that you start failing reps after your second set. Rather you want to find that perfect balance of struggling enough so that you only maybe miss a few reps in your last set.

More specifically...

When you're working on lower rep-ranges of 4-8 reps, MMF should be reached about one to two reps before your last set ends.

When you're aiming for higher rep ranges of 10-30 reps, you can fail anywhere between two and four reps before your last set ends.

So, let's say you wanted to do four sets of twelve repetitions of dips. If you start with twelve reps during your first set but the rest of your sets look something like this:

- ten reps for your 2nd set
- nine reps at your 3rd set and
- five reps at your 4th set

Then this means that you're going to failure way too early and too often.

On the other hand, if you start again with twelve reps during your first set and the rest of your sets look something like this:

- twelve reps for your 2nd set
- twelve reps at your 3rd set and
- ten or eleven reps at your 4th set

– you're spot on. For those who are beginner's and might have a bit of trouble figuring this out, don't worry. It can take some trial and error at first, but usually you'll get it right after a week or two.

Note: Make sure that once in a while you have someone experienced enough to check your form. It's easy to not be aware of some of your mistakes if you train alone long enough. Another way to do this is by recording your sets with a camera/your smartphone and reviewing your technique later.

Muscle-building Bodyweight Tip #1: Try to reach Momentary Muscle failure during your last 1-4 reps of each exercise's last set.

THE SCIENCE BEHIND TRAINING HARD & MUSCLE GROWTH

To better understand the importance of training till MMF, let's have a look at some basic physiology in regard to muscle recruitment. During any set you push yourself till failure, your nervous system will first recruit slow-twitch muscle fibers. When those are depleted, you begin to recruit fast-twitch muscle fibers. Lastly, when the force demands of the set cannot be met any more, your reach muscle-failure. But what are these slow and fast-twitch muscle fibers? I'm glad you asked!

Muscle-fibers are divided into slow twitch and fast-twitch. To understand this distinction imagine them as two different groups of workers. Think of the slow ones as skinny guys that have a bit more endurance but are not that strong. These are more engaged at low intensities and when you're doing those first repetitions of a set (before fatigue starts to build up). The faster ones are the more jacked dudes that come into play when the skinny guys cannot handle anymore the high intensity, explosive work and high mechanical tension. Unfortunately, these have less endurance, so they run out of steam faster.

In summary, the more you push yourself (the closer you get to MMF) or the more explosive work you do – the more of your fast-twitch muscle fibers are recruited. The reason this is important for muscle-growth is because fast-twitch fibers have a far greater growth capacity (about 50% more) than the slow ones!

For example, let's say I can do ten pull-ups if I push myself till MMF. This means that during the first three to four reps, I'm using more of my slow-twitch muscle fibers. Somewhere around the sixth or seventh rep, I struggle more and more to lift my body close to the bar. This means that the slow-twitch muscle fibers are almost completely fatigued, and my body begins recruiting more fast-twitch muscle-fibers. By the tenth rep, most of the muscle fibers (fast and slow) in my back and arms have been recruited and depleted. In other words, I'm too tapped out to get another rep. If I had not pushed myself hard enough and stopped around the sixth rep, I wouldn't have achieved a decent amount of fast-twitch muscle-fiber recruitment (hypertrophy).

Final thoughts on training hard...
Training hard is a skill... the more you practice it the better you get at it. Pushing yourself to the limits while maintaining good technique requires focus and embracing discomfort. This is not that easy to do since when your neuromuscular system is tapped, your body just wants to let go of the tension and relax. If you're a beginner don't let this discourage you, and don't beat yourself up if you're not good at it yet. The more you practice the better you'll become and the less uncomfortable you'll start feeling. It will become a sensation you learn to appreciate and even enjoy. Personally, the closer I push myself to my limits, the more satisfaction my workouts offer me. Of course, this is something I began appreciating through time.

CAN YOU BUILD MUSCLE WITH HIGH & LOW REP-RANGES?

Sticking between 8-12 reps was the typical advice for hypertrophy when it came to rep ranges during last couple of decades (especially in the bodybuilding community). Based on most of the latest research, it seems that mid-range reps might still have a slight edge over lower and higher reps when it comes to hypertrophy. However, recent studies, show that higher and lower rep ranges can be beneficial for adding muscle mass as well. When total load (reps X weight or intensity) are matched, lower and higher reps can be quite effective (if not equally effective) at building muscle. In simple words, everything works as long as you do enough of it and work hard at it.

Low reps

In the past, lower reps where thought to improve mostly strength (the ability to handle high intensity for about 1-5 reps) but not add that much muscle. That is why for example, people think that pro weightlifters can lift heavy weights without being that buff. In reality, it's not so much the rep ranges they use, but rather other things that have to do with their nutrition and sport. For example, a lot of them have to stay light since they have to compete at a specific weight category. Gaining mass when your caloric intake is limited is not possible after a certain point. What about those on the highest weight category then, you might think? Well, those guys are actually pretty big and muscular but... the reason their physique doesn't look that impressive is because they also have extra fat that covers things such as muscle-definition and vascularity. Heavyweight lifters don't care about looking lean – they care about lifting heavy things.

Another reason why pro weight-lifters' physiques don't look that impressive is because they don't work a lot on exercises that build prominent and aesthetic muscles, such as the chest and biceps. Instead of focusing on muscle tension, they use explosive and highly technical movement, lifting most of their loads with big muscle groups such as the back and lower body. Therefore, their biceps and pecs might not be that big but their backs and legs are usually quite ripped for their weight.

Practical implications for building bodyweight muscle with low reps

Using low reps, is unavoidable when you're trying to master challenging calisthenic exercises such as one-arm push-ups. Even more basic stuff like regular pull-ups take a lot of work for beginners. For example, let's say you haven't been able to do pull-ups yet. Working on easier variations with higher reps should be your main focus at first (i.e. do assisted band pull-ups). At some point you'll begin to do your first few reps with good form. This means that you'll be working on low-repetition sets (3-5 reps) for a while before you start getting closer to a more mid-range (6-8 reps).

During a low rep-range set, in order for our body to handle high intensity effectively, both slow and fast-twitch muscle fibers have to be recruited quite early. This improves the communication between your neuronal pathways and your muscle cells. Scientifically said: Low rep ranges improve motor unit activation (motor neurons integrated to muscle fibers). All this allows you to still progress in terms of gaining muscle while working your way up from low rep ranges to more optimal mid-ranges (aka body-building ranges).

Conclusion: Getting stronger is always useful for getting bigger...

High reps
High rep-ranges, meaning anything above sixteen repetitions, were thought to improve mostly muscle-endurance without increasing muscle mass that much. Although this is disproven, there a lot of people who still believe and perpetuate this theory. A typical example of this are women who train with light loads (i.e. pink dumbbells that are as heavy as a bottle of water) using high rep-ranges because they read in some magazine that this will tone their arms without making them too bulky. The reason these women don't gain muscle (besides the fact that gaining muscle comes a lot slower for women) is because they're not pushing themselves hard enough. In other words, it is not because of the high rep range, but because of not using enough of a challenging intensity that will cause muscle failure and fast-twitch muscle fiber recruitment.

In reality, the latest research has shown that as long as you train close to Momentary Muscle Failure (MMF), going as high as thirty to forty repetitions can be almost as effective as mid-rep-ranges are for hypertrophy.

Side-note: There is no such thing as toning! All you can do is simply add a little muscle (which is what most people mistake as toning) or gradually build a lot of it. When a client of mine tells me the typical "I don't want to gain too much muscle – I just want to tone my body" all I can do is smile and try to explain the above. I tell them not to worry since no one suddenly wakes up one day looking like a jacked Hollywood actor who is going to be in the next Superhero movie (which would be pretty awesome for most of us). In the end I let them understand that if they reach a point where they do not wish to add more muscle mass we can simply switch their program to maintenance volume and intensity.

Practical implications for building bodyweight muscle with high reps
Switching to high reps is a tactic I like to use once someone is past their intermediate phase and they need to switch things up a bit. This can be an especially useful strategy if you're experiencing hypertrophy plateaus. Working with high reps (i.e. doing sets of 20-30 reps) is usually not the best approach for beginners.

First of all, you're not strong enough to apply them in most exercises. For example, doing twenty perfect-form pull-ups takes years of practice for most people. Second, it might not be a favorable rep-range for many people since training close to muscle failure with high reps can be uncomfortable. Let's say you compare a set of eight reps and a set of thirty reps, both resulting in the same momentary muscle failure. With the thirty-rep-set, the burn you feel in your muscles builds up after about twenty reps or even earlier. This means that you have to withstand muscular discomfort for about ten reps. With eight-rep sets on the other hand, muscular discomfort will be more prominent during those last three reps.

Another consideration for people with limited time is that high-rep sets can make your workouts a bit longer, since your set duration doubles or triples.

Conclusion: High reps are great for hypertrophy once you reach a more advanced level.

Bodybuilding reps: Still the best approach
All the quality research up to this point continues to support that focusing on the traditional bodybuilding mid-rep range is essential for getting big. This makes sense since it's how the majority of people got big in the past. There's nothing magical about the 8-12 range. The reason it works is because it's long enough to produce an ideal balance between high intensity and metabolic stress in the muscle, which are both essential factors for muscle growth. High intensity leads to fast twitch muscle fiber recruitment, and metabolic stress is connected to storing additional muscle glycogen (in simple words - liquid muscle sugar). Glycogen is one of the fuels used by the muscles within this range, and it contributes to the increase of our muscle's size by supporting more muscle fiber growth.

I also consider this rep-range ideal for practical reasons. For starters, as explained in the previous example, it's an ideal time under tension to push yourself hard while focusing on perfect technique, and it keeps your workouts relatively short.

BODYWEIGHT EXERCISE ADAPTATIONS FOR BUILDING MORE MUSCLE

Working within that 4-12 rep-range is practical. As you get stronger though, you have to find a way to make exercises challenging enough. Remember, progressive is key in order to keep building muscle and improving your physique. Here is what you'll usually find people recommend when it comes to exercise variations and progressions:

- Changing the hand-stance for upper body exercises (i.e. wider or narrower hand-stance for push-ups, pull-ups or dips).
- Adding extra weight through weight vests, weight belts, etc.
- Doing single arm versions for upper body exercises (i.e. move from normal push-ups to one-arm push-ups).

Let's examine these options one by one...

One-arm bodyweight variations that are worth your time
One-arm variations that use full-bodyweight are not something I'd recommend to most people. For example, the one arm pull-up is considered the holy grail when it comes to bodyweight exercises and relative strength. After working on them for years, I managed to achieve one arm pull-ups for both my left and right arms. And although I've written and created extensive tutorials (you can find detailed blogpost on T-nation.com and a shorter video-version on my YouTube channel) I don't consider them useful for hypertrophy or for long-term bodyweight fitness.

For starters, unless you have a background in gymnastics or extreme relative strength, I find that it takes about ten to sixteen months to achieve a single one-arm pull-up with your strong arm/side for the average/semi-advanced trainee (someone training consistently with calisthenics for at least two years). It is something that takes serious methodical and consistent training. And that's just for getting one rep with your strong arm! Your weak arm can take up to double that time (it took me almost three years). Doing slow and clean one-arm pull-ups for reps is impossible for 99% of the population. Sure, there are some people that get the OAPU a lot faster than average and people who can do multiple reps, but these are simply the exception to the rule. If you do manage to get a couple of reps after a lot of practice, most likely they'll be done in a very explosive manner that doesn't allow you to focus on muscle contraction and hypertrophy.

Lastly and most importantly, it's a high-risk exercise when it comes to injury. Working on the OAPU can have you flirting with elbow inflammation and tendonitis in no time, no matter how careful you are. Especially for people with sensitive elbows and/or those above thirty years old, I'd say it's not worth the risk.

Just to be clear, I'm not saying you shouldn't train for the one-arm pull-up if your joints are young and sturdy, and if you feel like it could be a cool milestone in your bodyweight journey. I definitely enjoyed working on it myself and felt awesome when I achieved it. Just keep in mind what are your goals, priorities and the risk factors associated with everything you do when you train.

Nowadays I've stopped working on the OAPU since joint health and maintaining a long-term bodyweight fitness lifestyle are my top priorities. Especially for those on a tight schedule, such as students and people that have families and a full-time job – I find it best to make every training minute count.

One-arm Push-ups and One-arm Inverted Rows
The one-arm push-up and the one-arm inverted row are two of the few single arm variations that I see value in if you're an advanced bodyweight trainee. For example, the one-arm push-up is quite a feasible advanced one-arm progression with lots of benefits. First of all, it can be accomplished within a matter of one to three months, and second... it looks pretty damn cool! Not only does it build massive shoulders, triceps and the chest, it's also a killer workout for your obliques (side-abs). If you're wondering what your obliques have to do with one-arm-push-ups, that's good question. First of all, even basic push-ups activate your core since you're in a plank position. Maintaining that straight body-line is done to a big extent by your core. During a one-arm push-up though, your obliques also have to compensate for the lack of stability caused by leaning on one arm. To do this, they act as anti-rotary muscles. In other words, they contract in order to maintain the side of your missing arm from turning towards your leaning arm. Once you master thirty push-ups with clean form, I highly recommend working on progressions for the one-arm push-up.

You can also work on one-arm inverted rows. This is also great for activating the core, the lower body and balancing any discrepancies you might have in upper body pulling-strength.

Adding extra weight through weight vests, weight belts, etc.
Adding extra weight on bodyweight exercises can be efficient in terms of hypertrophy since it increases mechanical tension. But the question now becomes... are you still doing bodyweight training? Or has it turned more into weight-lifting? I'm not a bodyweight-zealot, neither am I advocating strict bodyweight exercise as the best workout method in the world. Hey, even I enjoy combining resistance bands and slam-ball tosses with my bodyweight routine every now and then. I do avoid weighted calisthenics as an integral part of my training though for two main reasons.

<u>Number one is joint health.</u> The more you load upper bodyweigh exercises with extra weight the more you risk joint inflammation. This is not really an issue if you're below thirty years old and you've had an active lifestyle growing up. Under these conditions, weighted calisthenics usually won't harm you and can help with strength and hypertrophy goals. But once you cross that biological threshold where your joints stop being as indestructible as they once were, things get tricky. Every extra pound you lift on top of your own bodyweight increases your chances for joint sensitivities. The most common problems are a) elbow pain from pull-ups, b) shoulder sensitivity from pushing exercises, and c) wrist pain from pushing exercises done with hyperextended wrists.

It's easy not to take these sensitivities seriously when they first show up. But... after years of observing many people, both online and at my local personal training practice, I've learned one thing for sure. Little aches and pains that are ignored and keep reappearing, eventually become chronic issues. Through time they get more and more difficult to treat and after a certain point too stubborn to completely get rid of.

The second reason I don't use extra weight is practicality. One of my goals with bodyweight muscle is to show people that everyone's gym can fit in an easy-to-carry around backpack. As long as you have a backpack with a set of gymnastic rings, a little yoga mat and a jump rope, nothing can stop you from getting a killer workout! You can train anytime and almost anywhere. You don't need a gym membership or special, expensive and heavy equipment.

The third reason why I like training mainly with my own body as a resistance, is that I can do it until I get old. As long as you pay good attention to all the advice and guidelines in this book, bodyweight exercise will keep your joints strong and injury free. Using targeted warm-ups (i.e. mobility drills), avoiding extremes, avoiding pull-ups with heavy weight-vests, using good form and having a plan that builds up intensity gradually are all crucial details for long term bodyweight fitness.

To conclude, this book won't focus on weighted calisthenics since I believe that there are other more practical, safer and equally efficient ways to increase intensity and hypertrophy. Still, the workout plans in this book can also be done with extra weight. So, before we change topic, here are some important tips for weighted-calisthenics enthusiasts: a) if you do add extra weight make sure that form is always clean, b) do slow reps without any bouncing and rough movement, c) use grips that allow your joints to move freely (i.e. do you pull-ups on rings) and are more anatomical for your *joints (i.e. do you push-ups with push-up-grips or on your knuckles)*.

Changing the width of your arm and leg-stance or hand-grip
Common variations such as wide hand-stances for push-ups or wide grips for pull-ups are used because they are thought to increase chest and lat activation. In reality, not only won't these variations increase chest and lat activation in each exercise, but they can even cause shoulder and back injuries. I talk about this extensively in my books "How To Build A Greek God's Chest With Push-Ups" And "How To Sculpt At Gymnast's Back With Pull-Ups". Narrower hand-stances for pushing exercises such as dips or push-ups, and narrower grips for pull-ups can also cause too much torsion in the joints, and lead to shoulder and elbow problems. Tweaks like these that are done in order to make exercises more challenging are not a smart move. Maintaining proper anatomical hand-stances, grips and general solid good form in all bodyweight exercises is important for maintaining healthy joints and connective tissues in the long run.

After all, there is a better and more simple way to make exercises more difficult...
Do less but harder reps...
Lifting weights or doing weighted calisthenics has the advantage of easily adjusting the intensity of each exercise. This might not be an option you have with strict calisthenics but do not worry. There is a way to replicate the effect weighted calisthenics have on

your muscles without having to use actual extra physical weight. You also don't have to make big changes in the way the exercise is performed. No need for weird wide hand-stances that mess-up your form and can cause injuries and joint sensitivities. Using Mind-to-Muscle-connection (MMC) techniques causes your muscles to contract harder – as they would if you were to add extra weight onto yourself. And the best thing is that they do this without extra stress for the joints.

The way you do this is by focusing on specific inner cues/sensations that allow you to consciously make your muscles contract harder. This increases neural activity, muscle-fiber recruitment and local fatigue. All this also results in greater hypertrophy! In summary, instead of doing more reps or using harder variations, you focus on making your current reps harder. Think of it like this... if your body is the barbell you lift during bodyweight training, MMC techniques are the way you can mentally add more weight onto that barbell.

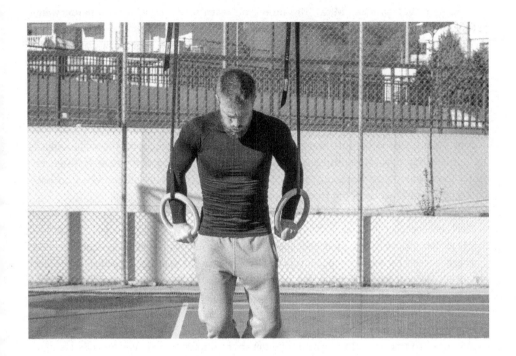

"If your body is the barbell when practicing calisthenics, MMC techniques are a mental way you can load your barbell."

~ *Bodyweight Muscle*

The more you practice MMC, the more you learn how to add more mental weight onto your barbell/body. This way you can make the exercise more challenging and keep on building muscle effectively while sticking at the same rep-range. In a way you learn how to command your muscles to work harder. It's a bit like a superpower! Well, maybe not a superpower that rescues people from burning buildings, but rather a training superpower you can use to naturally build more muscle. Still pretty cool, right?

An important distinction that must be made here is that MMC won't help you do more reps. On the contrary, applying MMC techniques will actually result in a decrease of reps. Again, this is because the goal of MMC is to make your reps more challenging. So, don't worry if you're doing less reps when you get started with these techniques – that's the whole point! It means you're doing it right. This way you can work on lower rep-ranges again, while doing the same exact exercise.

Once you've learned the basic external technique of each exercise, your next step is to start developing the inner technique. In other words, as you progress past the point of the beginner phase, your goal shouldn't just be doing more reps. It should also be learning how to do harder reps. You want to focus on increasing the intensity of each repetition by perfecting technique and contracting muscles consciously. To maximize your mind-to-muscle-connection, eliminate any excessive movement that doesn't help you increase muscle tension (i.e. using momentum, smaller ranges of motion, etc.). Training this way also gives more depth to your workouts. You learn to be more in the moment. As you get out of your head and get more into your body your mind also starts to calm down. You think less but you feel more. Remember... Don't just count reps – feel your reps!

Getting started with MMC

The exercises I recommend you start practicing MMC on are Pull-ups and push-ups. I highly recommend reading my books *"How to sculpt a Greek God's Chest with Push-ups"* and *"How to Carve Gymnast's Back with Pull-ups"*. By learning to apply MMC to one pulling and one pushing movement pattern you'll understand how MMC works for most exercises. Keep in mind that you should be able to perform at least twelve reps, with perfect form, in any exercise before your start applying MMC. MMC is about using perfect form, while utilizing your mind-to-muscle connection, in order to increase muscle contraction as much as possible.

One thing to keep in mind with MMC techniques is that although they're very effective for the upper body, they're not really that effective for the lower body. I wasn't completely sure if this was only my personal experience at first, but scientific research has also started to confirm it. The reasons are not clear yet but a hypertrophy researcher shared with me one speculation. He told me that it might have to do with the way our upper body and lower body differ in terms of sensitivity and their connection to the central nervous system. This is also one of the reasons why we take advantage of training methods such as plyometrics and sprints when it comes to the lower body.

Building lower body muscle with Plyometrics
Plyometrics (or jump-training if you prefer a more simple and self-explanatory term) are a very handy training method for challenging the lower body. Their advantage is that they force your muscles to contract more explosively, to produce close-to-maximum force in short intervals of time. Simple bodyweight exercises such as squats and lunges can become a lot more challenging by adding a jump at the end of the rep (aka jumping squats and jumping lunges). The more you strive for jumping higher, the more fast-twitch muscle fibers are stimulated and the more you increase fatigue. This also leads to more metabolic stress. As you've understood by reading this book so far, these are all ideal conditions for maximizing muscle-growth.

Building lower body muscle with Sprints
During high intensity anaerobic exercises such as thirty-second uphill sprints, your legs are forced to work hard enough that they come close to momentary muscle failure (MMF). This creates metabolic stress and causes your body to recruit fast-twitch muscle-fibers. The end result are muscular adaptations similar to those obtained from lifting heavy weights. Using plyometrics and uphill sprints strategically in your weekly routine will help you build strong, defined and muscular legs. These exercises are a lot more efficient than typical low intensity bodyweight exercises you see a lot of people wasting time on in the calisthenics routines (i.e. none-weighted bodyweight squats). Another bonus these exercises offer is that your core also gets a decent amount of activation from them.

In summary, Plyometrics and Sprints are the best bodyweight choice for building lower body muscle. They are short in duration and high enough in intensity to fatigue, they stimulate your muscles in depth and they successfully trigger hypertrophy.

Take away points of Bodyweight Rep-Ranges for Building muscle
In order to optimize muscle growth with calisthenics for the upper body, you want to focus on a middle muscle-building rep-range of ideally five to twelve repetitions. When you start advancing, a good way to stick to low/middle rep-ranges while keeping the exercises challenging enough, is taking advantage of MMC (Mind-to-Muscle-Connection) techniques. These are more effective for the upper body and take some practice but they can be an amazing supplementary weapon in your muscle-building arsenal. When it comes to the lower body, plyometrics (jumping-exercises) and sprints are the way to go once you move passed your beginner's phase. As you advance more and more, higher rep-ranges can be also helpful for breaking muscle-growth and physique plateaus.

The main rule to always remember is that you want to make sure you keep your sets challenging enough, by focusing on working close to MMF (Momentary Muscle Failure) while maintaining good form.

<u>Rep-evolution overview from beginner to more advanced</u>

1. *Master Basic Bodyweight Exercises:* Focus on getting at least a few reps with good technique for each bodyweight exercise. You can start as low as four reps.
2. *Work on increasing your reps:* Try to get to a point where you can perform about eight to twelve reps with most exercises.
3. *Focus on Mind-to-Muscle connection:* Don't just work on basic technique, focus on muscle contraction while executing the exercise with close to perfect form. Instead of more reps, try making each rep more challenging. This might decrease how many reps you perform since the intensity will increase.
4. *Plyometrics and Sprints:* For the lower body, the best way to increase intensity is adding a jump to basic squatting and lunging movement patterns. If you have the option, also add two sprint workouts to your weekly schedule. This is the best combo for building strong, athletic and muscular legs without any equipment.
5. *Specialized training methods:* Another way to increase intensity once you move passed your beginner's phase, are specialized training methods such as super-sets, circuits and rest-pause sets. These induce higher metabolic stress in order to challenge our muscles to grow more, by manipulating things such as exercise order and resting periods (more on these later as well).
6. *Add more Reps again:* As you start adjusting to higher intensities produced from the strategies above, start building up your reps again. Aim for eight to twelve perfect reps. Later on, even higher rep-ranges can helpful.

TRAINING VOLUME (HOW MUCH SHOULD YOU TRAIN?)

Training volume is the total amount of reps, sets and intensity that build up over a week. A key conclusion that research has made the last few years is that increasing training-volume as you progress over time is key for maximizing muscle growth. This means that besides quality (intensity and proper technique), quantity is also important. Once you move past your beginner progress (aka newbie gains), you have to start putting in more and more work if you want to keep advancing and breaking plateaus.

As shown in studies, there is a clear dose-response connection between training-volume and hypertrophy. One study showed that doing more than nine sets per week, per muscle-group, seems to produce almost twice the muscle growth compared to 5 sets per week. This doesn't mean that the more sets you do the merrier. There are limits based on your current level, and there are also specific strategies in the way you go by adding more volume.

This is why tracking your weekly training volume is key if you want to keep on building muscle and improving your physique as you advance. Small changes in training volume can help you see improvement when you're not seeing any progress for a while.

Muscle-building Bodyweight Tip #2: Track your weekly training volume

---

Measuring Training volume (prerequisites)
Simply going through the motions and banging more reps or sets to fill in your training log isn't enough for building muscle. I've probably repeated this a few times during this book already, but I'll keep on doing so since it's the core philosophy of Bodyweight Muscle. If you want your training volume to produce results, you need to make each set count by training focused and close to momentary muscle failure (MMF). Here are the standards that need to apply for a set to be included in your training volume:

a) *Proper warm-up:* Training-volume will always refer to the total number of sets done after a proper warm-up. Besides it being safer for your body, a proper warm up also increases performance.
b) *MMF:* Your sets should be challenging enough. Each set, should be on average, anywhere between 1-3 reps away from MMF.
c) *Proper form:* Your form should be close to perfect for all your reps. Avoid counting repetitions if your technique is bad. It is acceptable if during the last rep of your last set your form is a bit off due to over-exertion. But if during your sets, half of your reps are done with bad form, measuring training-volume will be pointless.

Calculating Training Volume (Movement over Muscle)
When it comes to weight-training, a functional way to calculate training volume is by measuring how much total weight per muscle group is being lifted per week. Let's say you do three sets of ten reps, during which you lift fifty pounds per rep – in total you've

lifted 3X10X50 = 1500 pounds. Multiply that by how many times you do this exercise per week and you have your total training volume. Although this can be applied to calisthenics, I do not find it practical nor in line with what calisthenics stand for.

Especially when it comes to bodyweight training, I believe that two people can lift the same weight for the same reps and have completely different results. As I've said, it's not just about reps but it's about focused reps: Being connected to your body and avoiding any excessive movement that cheats intensity from each repetition. While traditional bodybuilding breaks the body down to parts, bodyweight training should focus on the bigger picture – getting as strong as possible at essential movement patterns. This doesn't just build muscle, but it also develops an aesthetic bodyweight-kind of physique. Let's see which movements and which exercises related to these movements are the best for producing high intensity reps and building muscle.

1. **Pull:** The main targeted muscles areas here are Back and Biceps, and the best exercises to get started with are pull-ups and inverted rows.
2. **Push:** Main targeted muscles of this pattern are Chest, Shoulders and Triceps, and the best exercises to get started with are regular push-ups, pike push-ups and dips.
3. **Lower-body multijoint movements:** Main targeted muscles here – your entire lower body. The best exercises to work here are (for starters) basic squats and lunges, and later on jumping lunges, plyo-burpees and sprinting exercises.
4. **Movement (or resistance of movement) generated by the Core:** The core consists of your lower back muscles, your abdominals and the pelvic floor (the muscle that contracts if you try to pause peeing). It helps to think of this as whole when it comes to understanding exercise division in movement patterns, but for exercise selection you want to balance lower back targeted training and abdominal training. Best exercises here are planks, leg raises, hollow body, prone cobras and angels of death (more on these later on).

We'll talk a lot more about exercise selection and movement patterns further on in the book. For now, simply getting a basic understanding of all this is enough to understand how to organize your weekly training volume.

HOW MANY SETS FOR BUILDING BODYWEIGHT MUSCLE?

In comparison with rep-ranges, there is not a lot of research on set-ranges for hypertrophy (especially for bodyweight training). After a lot of trial and error during the last five years, I've managed to create a successful model regarding training volume dosages for building muscle with calisthenics. How did I end up with this model? Well, for starters I worked on combining and cross-referencing scientific literature with experiential evidence from the most successful coaches and bodybuilding athletes of the last century. During all this I also did a lot of personal testing and played with different methods and volume numbers. Sharing my results with my followers on BodyweightMuscle.com and HomemadeMuscle.com (my previous website) was another great way to gain feedback from many other bodyweight exercise trainees.

Lastly, training lots of people online and offline and seeing how their bodies reacted to my coaching style, was another helpful piece for putting together this puzzle. A cool thing about the internet is that it gives you the opportunity to cross-reference ideas with a large number of people really-fast – something we didn't have the opportunity to do in the past. This makes it a lot easier than it used to be to gather helpful data for research.

After five years of obsessing on Calisthenics Programming for building muscle I finally cracked the code! So, let's cut to the chase now and talk numbers…

Beginner's Training Volume: As a beginner calisthenics' trainee, during your first two introductory weeks, your minimum total weekly volume per Movement Pattern should be 8-9 sets. The following four weeks you can bump your training volume up to 12 sets and ideally spread them over four workouts.

Intermediate: The following twelve weeks you can move up to 12-14 sets per Movement Pattern. Ideal training frequency again here is four workouts per week. Three workouts per week also works pretty well for most people. What I don't recommend once you're passed your beginner phase is a two workout per week training frequency. Somewhere in the middle of this phase, it's a good idea to start introducing specialized training methods* to your programming.

Specialized training techniques stimulate hypertrophy by increasing metabolic stress. This is done through the combination of exercises (i.e. super sets) and manipulating resting periods (i.e. circuits). We'll talk a lot more about specialized training methods later in the book.

Advanced: Next, as you move from intermediate to advanced, you want to start working on 14-18 sets per movement pattern to get optimal results. Again, during this phase it's a good idea to challenge your muscles to grow through a combination of both the increased volume and specialized training methods.

Quick overview:

a) 9 sets per Movement pattern (first two introductory weeks)

b) 10-12 sets per movement pattern (next four weeks)

c) 12-14 per movement pattern combined with specialized training (next twelve weeks)

d) 14-18 + sets per Movement pattern combined with Specialized training (six to twelve weeks, alternated with maintenance/deload periods)

Note 1: Especially for the advanced phase, the training volume recommended is not meant to be performed consistently for more than 12 weeks. Rather, it's meant to be used at peaking periods that have to be alternated with maintenance periods. Deload weeks should also be included every 6 weeks of consistent training. More on this in the next paragraphs...

Note 2: The core fires up a lot during bodyweight exercises. Because of that, even half the volume of what you do for the rest of the movement patterns can be enough for core targeted movements. Other than that remember that abs are also made in the kitchen!

The numbers above are not meant to be set in stone. They're meant to serve you as guidelines and a reference point during your first year of training consistently with calisthenics. Some people with good genetics can tolerate even more volume, while others can sometimes benefit from trimming down their volume a bit. Once you start training consistently for more than a year, you'll learn to listen to your body better, and you'll be slowly able to start figuring out what works best for you. You'll figure out a personal minimum effective dose that stimulates hypertrophy. This should be a bit higher than your maintenance volume. When you adapt to that, you can always kick it up a notch by adding more volume and alternating specialized training methods. This is the only way to keep breaking through plateaus. Just remember as a rule of thumb, you don't want to be adding more than one set per week, and not less than one set per six weeks.

OVERREACHING AND SUPERCOMPENSATING

As I said earlier, training volume is important but that doesn't mean the more you do the better. You can't push the pedal to the metal the whole-year-round. Your body does have limits. Especially once you reach an advanced phase (meaning you have been training consistently for more than 18 weeks), you have to learn to alternate between high volume/intensity periods and deload weeks/maintenance periods. There are different systems to do this, but the general idea is the following:

a) You want to train more and more until your body is so tired that it's on the edge (or slightly crosses it) of underperforming. A slight decrease in your performance is ok, just don't overdo it.

b) After that, take a step back and reduce intensity and workload for a while. This will allow your body to fully recover and prepare you to handle the same or a little bit more hard work more efficiently the next time.

To rephrase this in a shorter and a bit more scientific way – you want to increase volume to a point of functional <u>overreaching</u>, after which you take a step back in order for your body to <u>supercompensate</u>. Let's have a brief look at what these two terms mean.

Overreaching is training with more stress/volume than what your body is used to, which gradually results in a decrease of your performance. This shouldn't be confused with overtraining, which leads to a loss of performance for longer amounts of time and can even cause health problems. Some people worry a bit too much about overtraining, when the reality is that they've barely ever gotten close to overreaching. Overtraining requires extreme amounts of training that are only possible for professional athletes.

Supercompensation is what can follow *overreaching* if you're strategic with your training. Once you reach a point of functional overreaching, it has to be followed by at least two days of complete rest (no training), and after that a few days of low intensity and low volume workouts. Giving your body the opportunity to recover at the right time, allows you to compensate above your previous capacities, and thus improve your ability to handle even more training stress/volume in the future.

Deload weeks

A good way to do this is with deload weeks. I recommend these once every five weeks, meaning for every five weeks of training consistently with the appropriate amount of training volume for your level – take a step back and have a deload week. During deload weeks, training frequency, intensity and volume can be reduced. There are multiple ways to do this but here is one I recommend: Drop training frequency down to two or three workouts per week (at least one workout less than previously). Cut your training volume in half and decrease your reps by twenty percent. For example, if you were doing ten pull-ups now go for eight. "Trisets" are also a great way to structure your workouts for intermediates and advanced bodyweight trainees. We'll explain these later on in specialized training.

Maintenance Volume

Even with the use of deload weeks, chronic high-volume training can desensitize your muscles to growth. This is why training at maintenance volume a couple of times per year is also important for muscle growth. Maintenance Volume (MV) is the minimum dose of training volume that allows you to maintain your current level of muscle mass. No matter how long and hard you train to reach a point where you're happy with your physique and strength, you still have to keep doing a specific amount of training to maintain those results.

Knowing your MV is also pretty handy when life is catching up and training as much as you'd like to is not always possible. During such times it can help you focus on the minimum amount of work you have to do in order not to watch your hard work go down drain. This way you can also give yourself a bit of slack when you need it, rather than beating up your already drained self with unnecessarily high expectations.

For example, I'm training at MV as I'm editing this part of book. This period has been probably the busiest of my life. I'm putting a ton of work into finishing the book you're reading, I'm preparing for a bodyweight training certification course I'll be teaching in Greece in three weeks, I'm working on improving the video production on my YouTube channel, I'm setting up a small Bodyweight training studio to train people indoors during the winter, I'm doing more personal training with clients, plus a bunch of other smaller stuff. Trying to make progress and train with an advanced workout plan right now would probably burn me out. So instead, I train four times a week, doing short volume and moderate to high-intensity workouts. My training is exactly enough to maintain my strength and muscle mass. It helps me take the edge off mental stress without draining me energy-wise. And, it is quite short so it doesn't take too much of my limited time.

Even if you might have to compromise with a bit lower volume than MV because you're going through an extremely busy period, it's still better than nothing. This might lead to a small decrease in muscle-mass, but thanks to muscle memory you'll build it back up in a matter of about ten to fifteen days once you start training more again.

> *Geeky science titbit:* Did you know that you have your satellite cells to thank for what is called muscle-memory? These special cells remain dormant at rest, but they're awakened by muscle contractions and muscle damage once you start training again with your regular routine. These cool cells are what help speed up muscle growth again.

It would be cool if after we reached our goal, we could train whenever we felt like it and maintain our results. Unfortunately, that's not how our body works. When it comes to our body's priorities, maintaining muscle mass is not very high on the list. If you're not motivating your physiology hard enough through adequate training volume and intensity, it will start getting rid of your hard-earned muscle pretty fast. What you want to remember is that the amount of work you have to put in to maintain your results once you reach a point you're happy with, is less than the work you had to put in to reach that point. Obviously for a beginner this amount is lower than what it is for a more advanced trainee. But nonetheless it's good to know that you can take it a bit easier. So how much work do you have to put in to maintain your progress? Although this can vary for advanced trainees, here are some general numbers that work for most people.

Sets per Movement pattern per week for maintenance:

- Beginners: 8 sets
- Intermediate: 10 sets combined with some specialized training
- Advanced: 12 combined with specialized training.

Keep in mind that training volume for advanced trainees might vary, since there are a lot of levels of how advanced one might become. Start with twelve sets and if you see that that's not doing the trick, kick it up a notch to about fourteen.

Some extra thoughts on maintenance and long-term fitness
Most people underestimate the work required to get advanced results and overestimate the work it takes to maintain them. Learn to be flexible and go with the flow of life. This can mean a lot of things, but I definitely don't mean it in a make-excuses-to-avoid-training kind of way... You'll have tough periods in life during which training hard will have the potential to help you get through that phase. But you'll also have periods when the demands will be high. Taking it a bit easier with your training, in order to focus on the current emergencies and priorities is the smart move during such times. Knowing the amount of minimum effort required to maintain what you've built up-to that point will help you with not having to stress about and over-think things such as "Am I doing enough?", "Am I failing on my fitness lifestyle?", "Am I a quitter?", "Is all my hard work going to waste?". Lastly, don't over-force yourself to train. Sometimes you need some distance from all your habits, even the good ones. Your bodyweight routine will be always there for you once you decide to get back at it.

TRAINING FREQUENCY

Minimum training stimulus of a movement pattern should be two times a week. The main reason for this is that exercise induced muscle-growth doesn't last more than three to four days after the workout. After that, your muscle begins to return to its original untrained state. A typical mistake I often hear from calisthenics trainees is applying the classic bro-split to the way they structure their weekly training. A bro-split based workout plan means that you train each muscle group once per week. This is a bodybuilding method that was promoted a lot by bodybuilding magazines, but it is one of the worst ways to structure your workout plan – either you're a calisthenics trainee or even if you work out at the gym.

How a typical Bro-split workout plan looks like:

1. Monday is chest-day (meaning you only train chest)
2. Tuesday is back-day (you only train the back)
3. Wednesday is leg-day (...you get the deal)
4. Thursday is arm and ab-day
5. Friday is shoulder-day.

Here's what happens when you train a muscle-group/movement pattern one time per week... The first three to four days after your workout, you'll have adaptations that lead to increased strength and muscle size. After resting for more than that though, the targeted muscle-group begins returning to its initial state. This happens because there is no new stimulus to sustain the new adaptations. In other words, there is not accumulation of training volume and stimulus to induce or maintain muscle growth. Training a muscle group less than twice a week might work a bit only if you're a beginner (which is when even really small amounts of training can produce results) or if you have amazing genetics. It also works if you use illegal substances such as steroids that elevate muscle-growth for more than four days, which was the reason that bodybuilders promoted this type of training.

Muscle-building Bodyweight Tip #3: Don't train a movement-pattern less than twice a week.

After you've made sure that you train each movement pattern two times per week, training frequency (TF) depends on how you want to spread your weekly training volume. For example, stuffing all your training volume in two weekly workouts is doable when you're a beginner and training volume is low. As you progress and training volume increases, it's a good idea to also increase TF in order spread your training volume a bit more over the week.

Can you train every day?
I wouldn't recommend training every single day of the week. Training six days per week though can be both doable and effective. I wouldn't recommend training every single day of the week though. Technically it can work but the main reason I recommend not it is more psychological that physiological. Breaking your daily patterns at least once a week is important for maintaining those same habits. Taking a rest day, besides recharging you physically, will also recharge you mentally.

High frequency training allows you to do short duration but high intensity workouts. This is handy for advanced trainees that have a lot of volume to handle. High training frequencies can also be handy for busy people that like to train on a fixed daily schedule. Your workouts feel more automated that way, and it can be easier to remain disciplined. If this sounds like it makes sense to you, you can give it a try. For complete beginners who are interested in a high-frequency training schedule, I recommend starting with 3 workouts per week during your first two weeks to allow your body to gradually adapt. After that you can move on to a six-workout-per-week frequency.

In summary, as long as movement patterns and sets are spread in a balanced way across the week, training almost every day is not only doable – but it can be even more effective and practical for some people. Think about it and see what fits your lifestyle best.

HOW LONG SHOULD YOU REST BETWEEN SETS?

Typical bodybuilding training guidelines used to recommend short rest intervals of about thirty to sixty seconds for maximizing muscle growth. This was based on the premise that higher metabolic stress associated with limiting rest between sets promoted a greater muscle-building stimulus.

Current research has shown that longer resting periods are superior to shorter ones. For example, here's what one study showed in people lifting weights when comparing three minutes to one minute of rest. Those who rested three minutes had a logical increase in performance. It makes sense that you have more strength in your next set when you rest more... Secondly and most importantly, they also had an increase in muscle thickness. Although it's not yet known why this happens, leading researchers in the field of hypertrophy speculate that it's probably attributed to the increase of total intensity and training volume produced by doing more reps or lifting more weight. The same goes for bodyweight training. The more you rest, the more quality repetitions you can perform in each set.

The conclusion here is that very short rest periods may compromise growth by reducing the number of reps and intensity you can handle on subsequent sets. I always thought that resting enough in order to perform well on each of your sets was very important for muscle growth. Now that there's research confirming it, I'm convinced of the value that long resting periods have for hypertrophy.

That is not to say that short breaks are bad. It just means that it's not an ideal long-term resting strategy. There is a time and a place for short breaks. Like, for example, when you're using specialized training methods (i.e. supersets and circuit training). Also, if you're short on time it's better to have short resting periods than missing out on part of your workout. Again, it's a matter of what's optimal and what's functional for you. If you can, it's best to get enough rest between sets during most of your workouts.

As Brad Schoefeld says (leading researcher in strength training and hypertrophy): *"if there are synergistic benefits to heightened metabolic stress in short resting periods, they are overshadowed by the associated decreased volume."*

Practical applications for Calisthenics

So how does this apply to bodyweight exercise? When you're working with hypertrophy oriented rep-ranges (6~12 reps), a good general recommendation would be resting two to three minutes. Some people recover a bit faster than others. Therefore, two minutes will do it for them. Other people recover slower so they might gravitate more towards the three-minute threshold. When you're training outdoors and in low temperatures make sure you stay active during your resting periods. Personally, I like to walk in between sets. Especially when training in cold temperatures, avoid going higher than three minutes of rest since your body will start cooling off and you'll need to re-warm-up.

Another thing to keep under consideration when it comes to your resting periods, is what kind of exercise we are talking about. For example, high-intensity multi-joint exercises, such as pull-ups and Handstand Push-ups, create large amounts of stress and are very taxing on the neuromuscular system. Because of this, it makes sense to rest at least two minutes between sets. Personally, when it comes to these kind of exercises, I'll take two minutes of rest during my first sets and up to three minutes for my last set. That way I'm sure that I'm rested enough and that I'll get as many reps as possible.

Resting periods also depend on the type of exercises performed. Exercises that are less metabolically taxing (i.e. most core exercises) can be done with resting periods as short as one-minute. This way, you can increase metabolic stress (and its potential hypertrophic benefits) without negatively impacting volume load. Ideally leave these exercises for the end of your workout, to ensure that they don't interfere with your recovery from highly taxing multijoint exercises. It's also a good idea to keep your core fresh in the beginning of the workout – especially for challenging upper bodyweight exercises where the core plays an important role for overall performance.

Considerations for Beginners: Another category of people that can save time through shorter resting periods without compromising performance are beginners. Most beginners don't have enough experience to know how to stress their body hard enough. As we said, training hard is also a skill. This is why I recommend short one-minute breaks in the beginner's phase. At least for the first eight to twelve weeks of training.

Considerations for advanced trainees: Although I agree that focusing on long resting periods is optimal for hypertrophy, I also believe that advanced trainees need a bit more variety in their training program. This is why I consider it valuable to incorporate short resting periods once or twice a week as an advanced trainee. Specifically, if you train three to four times per week, include one workout with short-resting periods. If you train five to six times a week you can incorporate up to two workouts with short-resting periods.

How to maximize recovery:
Resting periods aren't meant for you to login to your Facebook with your mobile device to catch up on your notifications. Try to fully focus on relaxing your whole body and especially the muscles that are tensed. Whether you're aware of it or not, even while resting between sets you're still producing slight amounts of tension. The reason you don't observe this is due to the contrast between high muscle tension during your set and lower muscle tension during your rest. Let's take pushups for example. After completing a set, observe how you might be still keeping your shoulders and neck a bit tight.
Try observing yourself by scanning your body up and down one time. Look for tensed areas, these will usually be very common. For me and many other people, these are typically the shoulders and the neck/upper trapezius. Others might be unaware they are squeezing their fists or jaw. Resting actively by walking a bit around while relaxing your body, allows your neuromuscular system to recharge a bit faster.

Summing it all up...

To fully optimize muscle growth, take advantage of long recovery periods (2-3 minutes). This will ensure that you recover adequately and that you aim for maximum training volume and intensity across sets. If you're on a tight schedule, it's ok to keep your breaks short of course. Just try not to go lower than one minute.

PART 2: NUTRITION FOR BUILDING BODYWEIGHT MUSCLE

When I first started writing this book, I wasn't sure if I should include nutritional information in it. But, since building muscle depends so much on having a proper diet, I decided to devote a Part to this topic. I wanted to make sure that none of my readers who put in the hard work would lack results because of nutritional mistakes.

This Part is not about giving you a detailed fixed nutritional plan to follow. Rather, it's about making sure you are covering all the basics when it comes to fueling your workouts. Just like with exercise, there is also a lot of contradictory information regarding nutrition. Before you start following any nutritional plan or weird diet – first be sure that you know how to cover all your basic needs and stay healthy in the long run. Again, just as with your training, your diet should also be part of your lifestyle – not something you do every now and then. In the end you'll learn that once the basics of your diet are set, the only thing you really need to tweak are your calories.

I've done most of the popular diets out there. I like to experiment with anything that is workout or nutrition related before I start criticizing it. I've been a vegetarian for half a year and I've also done paleo for a couple of months. I've tried a lot of fasting diets, I've done food-combining diets and a bunch of other diets that I don't even recall anymore. What usually happens with diets, is that we try them for a limited amount of time, and then we switch back to our previous nutritional habits. And because they'll often work for that limited amount of time, we'll think "hey, that was a good diet, why did I stop it?" I'm guilty of doing this multiple times in the past. The first thing you want to understand when it comes to nutrition is the following: If a diet is impossible to sustain in the long run – it's not a good diet (for you at least).

When I started Paleo for example, I experienced a big energy boost. I felt great and got pretty lean. I was eating and even sleeping less, I was training more and I felt unstoppable. At first, I thought it was because of the type of foods I was eating. Later on though, I realized it was because I was on a calorie deficit. This elevated my catecholamine levels, also known as the ''flight or fight response'' hormones. Some of these hormones, like adrenaline, noradrenaline and dopamine, can increase muscle strength, mental alertness and even produce a feeling of euphoria. For a limited amount of time, your body can increase catecholamines when you're restricting calories. This primal mechanism that keeps us in "hunting mode" when energy supplies are low. Mystery solved.

Later on though, my body started adjusting to the diet's effects, and I realized it wasn't a diet I could sustain long-term. After a certain point I needed more carbs to train efficiently, but also not be cranky. Yup, a lack of carbs can also mess up your mood... Plus, what's the point of living when you can't have some ice-cream on a hot summer day, or an extra-large pizza with your girlfriend while watching a good movie once in a while? You can still have those every now and then and look great. It's all about balance...

UNDERSTANDING HOW DIETS WORK

The truth is that every diet works. Well, at least the most popular ones (that's why they're popular). Diets simply help you feel better or lose weight by tricking you into eating less. What do I mean? Let's take Paleo diet again as an example. Paleo cuts out most carbs, sugar and processed food, which means that you can only eat food categories like meat, nuts and fruits. One problem with this diet approach is that it's really difficult to fill all your caloric needs based on these few high-satiating food categories - trust me I've tried! No wonder people "miraculously" lose weight on it. If you're overweight, it is something that can work for a while. At some point though, you will end up with low energy. Indulging in huge binge eating episodes every other week is something that happens pretty often to people who engage is such restrictive diets. This can even lead to serious eating disorders. Another trick Paleo and other diets use to help you eat less, is encouraging you to eat more protein. Protein has shown to be the most satiating macronutrient. This means that eating high-protein foods helps you feel full for longer periods of time, which again helps you eat less. Maybe Paleo is a good temporary solution for losing weight. But, if you want to gain muscle (which will require periods of being in a caloric surplus) it's definitely not the way to go.

Let's also examine an opposite type of diet like veganism. Vegan diets help a lot of people lose weight because they exclude two other major food categories, meat & dairy. At the same time, they also encourage you to eat more fiber, water and total food volume that is low in calories. Once again this is a good strategy to lose weight but once again a strategy that works only temporary for most people.

There is nothing wrong with strategies that help you regulate your weight. But, it's also important to make sure that these strategies are not causing you any nutritional deficiencies and unhealthy eating behaviors in the long run. People who follow extreme diets tend to have binge eating episodes and big fluctuations in their bodyweight (losing a lot, regaining a lot, etc.).

In summary, all diets work because they trick you intro controlling your calorie intake in some way. Fasting diets have you eating inside of a restricted window of time. High protein/low carb diets have you decreasing or removing carbs completely. Plant based diets increase the intake of low calorie and high-volume foods. Etc....

One of the reasons there is so much confusion out there with dieting is you. Yes, I'm talking about you, the person reading this book right now. Ok, it's not just you... it's also me and almost every human being with an internet connection looking up diet advice online. When it comes to dieting, we all prefer the easy way out. An article titled something like "TOP 10 FAT LOSS HACKS YOU AREN'T DOING" is going to have a way higher click-through rate than "Read this five-page detailed article to learn the basics of how to structure a healthy and sustainable diet". Remember... The fact that a diet works, doesn't mean that it's also sustainable!

If you want to succeed with your diet, you have to create a diet you can both enjoy and stick to. This doesn't mean that your diet should be always super easy, or that there won't be even short periods in your life that you mess it up a bit. In general though, creating a healthy proper diet plan requires discipline and being organized. You must find an approach that works for YOU.

Side-note: this part has nothing to do with food-ethics, I'm approaching nutrition here strictly from a general health and performance angle. If you're a vegan or vegetarian, I respect your choice from a moral standpoint.

BASIC RULES OF A PROPER DIET FOR
BUILDING MUSCLE & STAYING HEALTHY

As I've mentioned so far, a proper diet should primarily follow some basic rules. These rules should ensure that your body is getting enough nutrition for you to be healthy as you set muscle-building goals. In the following pages, I'll have you track things such as your calories and protein intake. Don't worry though, you're not going to have to do this for the rest of your life. Even though counting calories is the most effective weight-controlling strategy, it's also one more strategy that is not sustainable for most people in the long run. You'll only have to do this for a week. The pyramid below illustrates the three most important layers of every nutritional plan.

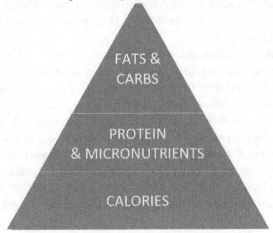

CALORIES COME FIRST

If you've read enough "best-selling" diet books, you've probably read things such as: how hormones can be manipulated through your diet to cause more fat loss without decreasing calories; how toxins are the reason you're not as lean as you'd like to be; how specific foods are the reason you don't have a six-pack; and all kinds of non-scientific or over-blown theories like that.

Unless you belong to that one percent of people that have special physiological problems (i.e. thyroid issues) things are pretty simple. The reason you're not losing fat or not gaining weight is that you're either eating too much or not eating enough. Sure, there are strategies that can help you optimize things. But, if you want to gain weight and the calories you get from food are less than the calories you burn – it doesn't matter how many protein shakes you drink. Or, if you want to lose weight and you are eating more calories than your body is burning – it doesn't matter how healthy you're eating or what special food your diet includes. There is numerous of solid scientific research on this topic and the conclusion always remains the same – if you eat more calories than you burn you'll eventually gain weight, just as if you eat less calories than you burn you'll eventually lose weight.

Counting calories and protein intake

As I said counting calories is something you have to do temporarily. I know it's boring... but be patient for a week. Think of how many hours we spend doing things such as watching tv shows or procrastinating on YouTube. I think we can all spare a couple of minutes a day for our health and exercise goals.

Here are some of the benefits of tracking your food intake...

1. Learning about nutrition: Tracking your calories will help you get a better understanding of nutrition. Things such as which foods are high in protein, which foods are rich in calories without being that filling (and the opposite), etc.
2. Eating more responsibly: People who know how to monitor their caloric intake effectively make more conscious eating choices and maintain a more stable weight in the long run. This is crucial once you build enough muscle and reach a weight you're happy with.
3. Flexibility: Tracking your calories allows you to even eat some of the forbidden /unhealthy things. As long as your calories are targeted to your goal and you get a decent percentage of your nutrition from whole foods, a little indiscretion here and there not only isn't a problem, but it can even support your goals.

The biggest problem for people wanting to gain weight and people wanting to lose it is the following: *Most people who want to lose weight underestimate how many calories they get (even nutritionists as shown in studies!) and most people who want to gain weight overestimate the calories they eat.* Tracking food intake for a week will allow you to be able to eye-ball your portions later on, and make better estimates of your caloric and protein intake. This will give you a tangible baseline to work from. There are plenty of tracking apps and websites out there that can help you keep track of your calories and protein. My favorite one currently is Loseit.com. You can log into their site, fill in your details and start tracking everything within ten minutes.

If you want to lose weight, aim at losing half to one percent of your total bodyweight per week. If you want to gain weight and muscle aim again for half to one percent of your total bodyweight per week.

PROTEIN INTAKE AND MICRONUTRIENTS

Protein is the building block of muscle, and together with fat these are the most essential macronutrients for your health. You can survive without any carbs but not without protein. If you're serious about your muscle-building goals, being aware of this macronutrient's daily intake in your diet is a must. Try to eat a variety of meat in your weekly schedule, preferring meats like fish & poultry over red meat. Avoid processed meats like hot dogs and bacon.

Good protein sources for omnivores:

- Lean meats (lean beef, poultry and any quality meat you can get)
- High protein dairy such as cottage cheese, Icelandic yogurt and Greek yogurt
- Eggs (ideally from grass-fed chickens)
- Fish (tuna, salmon etc)
- Whey protein (a scoop or two of whey protein per day can be handy for keeping your protein high when your dietary protein intake is low)

Protein sources for vegans/vegetarians:
- Grains and legume combos: Grains and legumes are called complementary proteins because when you combine them you get all of the essential amino acids you need to build muscle effectively. Rice and beans are an excellent example.

- Nuts and seeds, and combinations of them with legumes: Raw nuts, seeds and things such as hummus (chickpeas and tahini).
- Tofu, tempeh, and soy alternatives
- High protein dairy (for vegetarians) such as cottage cheese, Icelandic yogurt and Greek yogurt

How much protein do you need to build muscle with calisthenics?
0.7 grams per pound of bodyweight is a good start. If you can go for as high as 1 gram per pound of bodyweight even better. For example, if you're a guy who weighs 165 lbs then: 165 X 0.7 = 115.5 grams of protein per day is the minimum amount you want to be getting.

Protein intake adjustments for heavier than average people
Normally, the best way to set a protein intake is to calculate protein per pound of lean mass. A problem with this approach is that figuring out your lean mass is both costly and hardly accurate (all body-fat calculation methods have big discrepancies). Counting grams per bodyweight is effective for those with a relatively normal weight. For obese people though (over 20% body-fat for males and over 30% body-fat for females) you need to make special adjustments. For this population, going with 0.5 – 0.6 g per pound of body weight works better.

For example, if someone is 250lbs, an intake of one gram of protein per pound of bodyweight would mean that you need 250g of protein. This amount of protein is excessive and unnecessary. Using and adjusted intake of 0.5 – 0.6g of protein per pound seems to work well for this population.

Especially when losing weight, getting enough protein is crucial for your physique. When you're in a calorie deficit, besides burning your fat reserves you can also burn muscle. Yup, your body cannibalizes your own muscles. There are two ways to minimize this: One of them is strength training and the other is getting enough protein. Another reason protein is important on a caloric deficit is satiety. Protein is more satiating than either fats or carbohydrates. This is very helpful when calories are low and hunger is inevitably high. Protein will help keep you full and go through the process.

Micronutrients (Veggies & Fruit)
Whether you're a fan of them or not, you know that you need to eat your veggies every day. Try to include a colorful variety of them in your weekly schedule. The ideal intake per day is 4-6 portions. If you're not a fan, start with 1-2 portions per day and build it up to at least four portions. A veggie portion can be the equivalent of a cup, or your fist if you want a more personal analogy. You can't go wrong with veggies so don't worry about precise portions. Just eye-ball your portions fast and try to eat enough of them!

Note: Yes, there are some veggies with a bit more calories than average such as peas, but I don't think anyone ever got fat overeating boiled peas...

If you're eating enough veggies to cover your micronutrient needs, then three or even two portions of fruit per day can be enough. Not that its bad to eat more of them if they fit your daily caloric needs of course. A portion of fruit would be the equivalent of a medium-sized apple. Imagine the same size for most fruits. For example, if you're eating berries imagine how many berries would be required to fill the skin of an apple. Or for something more personalized imagine a fist again.

CARBS AND FATS

Once calories and protein intake are set you can let carbs and fats balance themselves self out based on your preferences. Find a balance that suits your lifestyle and taste preferences. Remember though, it's especially important to get enough healthy fats, since your body needs them for optimal hormone regulation and health. For example, a chronically low-fat diet can affect testosterone levels negatively, which will affect muscle growth as well.

As for carbs, they may not be *essential* to our survival (unlike protein and fats, we could survive without consuming carbs), but there's a difference between 'surviving' and 'thriving'. Plenty of carb-based foods contain important vitamins, minerals, fiber and are also important for regulating your mood.

How Clean should your diet be?
First of all, lets define what clean foods are. They are preferably home-cooked and minimally processed foods, such as fruits, vegetables, lean meats, rice, potatoes, and dairy. Ideally you want to avoid frying your food too long (stir frying veggies is ok), and choose cooking methods such as boiling, steaming, broiling, grilling, poaching, pressure-cooking or no cooking (raw).

If you're aiming at losing weight, stick to 90-95 clean eating. If you're aiming more at gaining weight, 80% will do. I'm not the obsessive clean-eater type and neither should you be. There's a place and time for most kinds of food.

The problem with non-clean foods is that they trigger overeating behaviors. For example, it's a lot easier to consume 1000 calories through donuts than through boiled potatoes. Give me a bucket of MnM's and a good movie and I'll keep eating them until I feel sick. By the way, keep in mind that for some people there are also "clean" foods that can trigger such behaviors. In which case even those should be limited. Keep foods that you have trouble controlling yourself with out of the house. This is especially important when you're trying to lose weight. The more temptation around you, the more likely you are going to drain your discipline resources and mess up your diet.

When can I have my "dirty" calories?
This depends on the person. Everyone's personal idiosyncrasies should be always taken into consideration when structuring a diet. For example, some of us don't like to have a small treat every day and would rather cash in all our cheat calories in the weekend. Others are fine with having a small portion every day. My tip for the second group is to have your cheat meal at the end of the day. It's easy to go downhill on a sweet/junk-food binge when you start your day with these kinds of foods.

Train for a better shape and diet for definition
As they say "you can't out-train a bad diet". Don't expect to get abs just by training hard enough. Sure, your training will give your abs muscle density, but unless you have your diet in control your abs will remain hidden beneath belly fat. Pull-ups will give you a wide back and muscular arms, but your diet will determine how defined your back and arms look. Did you know that an average workout doesn't burn more than 400 calories which is less than two slices of pizza? So, remember to train for muscle and diet for definition.

Weight-gain and Fat-loss plateaus
Whether you want to gain or lose weight, when starting your diet stick to it, even if you're not seeing any results for the first month. Sometimes the body takes time to 'catch up' with change. You need to give it enough time so you can have a clear idea of what's going on. After following your diet strictly for a month, here are some adjustments you can make if your weight gain/loss has come to a halt, or if you haven't experienced any changes at all.

Weight-gain tips
1) Eat 10-20% more with every meal: If you aren't seeing any progress after a month of following all the advice given to you so far, try eating 10 - 20% more than you regularly eat with every meal. Remember that your body is constantly trying to maintain homeostasis. This means that even if you focus on eating more calories around breakfast and lunch, you may unintentionally reduce your caloric intake during dinner without realizing it. This is a typical mistake hard-gainers make – they overeat during one or two meals, and don't realize that they're decreasing their calories during the rest of the day's meals (or even skip one or two). If you're doing this, you're just making a hole in the water that will leave you at calorie maintenance (or even deficit). So, focus on eating

10-20% more during all meals, instead of adding 30% to your lunch and eating 15% less during breakfast and dinner.

By gradually increasing your calories you can train your body to get used to eating more. You might need to force yourself a bit in the beginning, later on though, hunger levels will increase naturally. Eating at consistent times also helps with this. Ghrelin, also called the hunger hormone, controls when you get hungry. Eating at set times keeps Ghrelin consistent and creates consistent hunger patterns. This way you get hungry at similar times in the day and you can make sure you keep up with your increased food-intake.

2. Eat more healthy fats: Foods such as peanut-butter, virgin olive oil, high-fat Greek yogurt, etc., are great ways to sneak in a lot more calories in your daily eating schedule without stuffing yourself too much. Making shakes and smoothies with these foods makes it even easier to consume. There are tons of recipes you can find online. Just search for something like "healthy weight-gain shake".

3. Have snacks between meals: Nuts are a healthy, calorie-dense food that can easily increase your caloric intake. Make sure you have a minimum of a handful per day. Peanut butter n' Jelly sandwiches are another example. They're a fun and easy snack to add to your daily eating plan. Easy to make and carry with you as well.

4. Don't skip/forget meals: Eat a minimum of three big meals a day: Breakfast, lunch and dinner.

5. Have a badass dessert at the end of the day: As we said you can have up to 20% of "dirty" foods when gaining weight. This is about 500 – 700 calories (depending on your weight) you can cash in on a daily basis. My favorite cheat meal is chocolate, since it also has a decent amount of minerals, protein and vitamins instead of being empty nutrition like other desserts.

Fat-loss plateaus
1) Reduce calorie intake by another 5-10%: I.e. if your starting calorie intake was 2000 calories, you'd reduce it by another 100-200 calories. It's important to remember that as you lose fat, weight and become leaner, your caloric intake also decreases. This means that your caloric deficit must increase for you to continue to lose weight.
2) Increase NEAT: Something very important and yet neglected for fat-loss is total movement per day. NEAT is *Non-Exercise Activity Thermogenesis* which means that it is all your activity that isn't intentional exercise, such as walking, going up and down stairs, etc. NEAT is one of the most underrated tools for fat loss. We usually depend too much on burning calories through exercise instead of NEAT. Here's the thing though, exercise

is only one hour out of your day (and less for most people), which is about 5% of your day. Being more active throughout the day, such as walking or cycling instead of talking the car, taking the steps instead of the elevator – are all things that can add up in the end of a month. A really simple way to do this is to aim for ten thousand steps per day. There are special watches such as pedometers, that you can use to keep track of this. You can also simply download a phone app if you don't mind carrying your phone with you all day.

This is also one of the reasons peoples' diets stops being effective after a certain point. When you're on a diet for a while you'll tend to start moving around less since low calories can lead to decreased energy and increased lethargy. Therefore, tracking your daily movement is something to keep in mind during weight plateaus.

3) Weigh yourself daily: You want to do this in the morning, after using the bathroom and before eating breakfast. Because your weight can fluctuate day to day, it's important to keep track of your weekly averages over time in order to have a better picture of how your weight changes.

Dieting and exercise are a form of stress on the body. The longer you diet, the more this stress increases. The mental aspect of depriving yourself from foods and drinks you like doesn't help either with mental stress. So, when overall stress is elevated for a long period of time, cortisol (stress hormone) increases as well. As a result, you can begin retaining water. This water retention tends to be more prominent among women. Water retention can mask fat loss, and trick you into assuming you're not losing fat even in a calorie deficit, or worse, it can make you think you're even gaining weight. But if you stay patient enough, out of the blue, sudden magical flushes of weight can occur.

One thing that can help with this is taking 1-2 weeks off the diet and increasing calories up to maintenance. Increase calories mainly through healthy carbs. The reason I choose carbs is because they're connected to your mood. Done strategically this way, as a short break, carbs can make you happy. Meanwhile focus more on training hard. This will help reduce stress and drop water.

Maybe you're just Gaining Muscle

The scale is only one tool you should be using to track fat-loss. When your weight is not going down but body measurements, progress photos and strength improve... your body's ratio of fat to muscle is also improving. This means you're slimming down even though you're not losing weight.

For example, if you're a guy and your chest, arms, and quads measurements have increased while your stomach measurements have decreased, you're doing a pretty good job. You're probably gaining muscle and you're looking stronger and leaner. Ask people around you, I'm sure they'll agree.

Since we all enjoy fast and easily applicable tips, here are four you can try out for your fat-loss as well:

1.*Eat until 80% full*: Japanese call this *Hara Hachi Bu*. It simply means to leave the table without getting stuffed. The moment you feel your "tank" is 80% full, put down your fork/knife/spoon and leave the table. Learning to live with a balanced amount of hunger is key when you're looking to lose weight in a healthy and sustainable way. Whenever that feeling of tolerable hunger is present, don't think that you're hungry – think that fat-cells are protesting because they are slowly dying. If you struggle with this tip, applying the next one in addition, will make it a lot easier.

2. *Brush your teeth:* After applying hara hachi bu, get up from the table and brush your teeth for 3 minutes (minimum). I promise this will make it a lot easier, since the brain gets the message that your meal is over. It also increases your awareness. Having a clean mouth makes you think twice before you go on snacking again. If at some point this tip starts losing it's effect (might happen after a few weeks), also add teeth-flossing for 3 minutes after brushing your teeth. These tips might sound weird, but you'll be amazed by how effective they can be if you apply them. Just give them a try!

3. *Sequential eating:* Eat veggies or fruit at the beginning of each meal. Follow that by your protein-based food and leave your carbs for the end of the meal. This eating-order helps you reach satiety a lot faster and helps you eat more consciously.

4. *Replace your breakfast with a protein shake:* People think that breakfast is the most important meal of the day, something dispelled by modern science nowadays. If you don't feel really hungry during your first 3-5 morning hours, you can replace breakfast with a protein shake or simply fast. After that, go on with your daily routine by moving your 1st meal of the day 3-5 hours later. This will decrease your eating-window, allowing you to eat larger meals, which in turn will help keep you full, both mentally, and physically. One thing to watch out for with this tip in the beginning is to avoid overeating during your first meal. Hunger will be probably elevated during this meal from all the fasting, but through time you'll adjust.

5. *Coffee:* For a lot of people, coffee can suppress appetite. Try having a cup of black coffee instead of binging on unhealthy food, or if you want to delay having a meal a bit more.

Muscle-building Supplements supported by Science
There are very few supplements that actually work. Before you consider these, make sure that diet, training, and lifestyle are in order. If your diet and lifestyle are perfect,

supplements may add another 5% to your muscle building goals. Personally, although I am not anti-supplement, I usually find it too boring to deal with most supplements in my daily schedule, and I just prefer eating and spending money on real food. The main supplement I'll use from time to time is whey protein.

1. Protein Supplements: Increased protein consumption has been proven to aid athletic muscle building goals. Do you need protein powder for this? The answer is no. You can get all your protein through your diet if you want, and it makes no difference if you take no protein supplements. The reason protein supplements are helpful is because they are practical. Not everybody can eat a ton of meat and other protein rich food sources on a daily basis. We have busy schedules, we don't always have the luxury of cooking our meals, and finding proper sources of protein when eating out is not always possible.

For a lot of us protein can be also very costly. For example, in the Netherlands where I lived for a couple of years, quality meat was extremely expensive. A scoop of quality protein cost less than 1 euro/dollar when getting the same grams of protein could cost me quadruple that price. Back then, when funds were low, it was more realistic and practical for me to supplement my protein intake through whey protein. I don't mean you should substitute your dietary needs with supplements. But you also need to do the best with what you've got at times. If you can afford it, by all means get all the quality protein you can. Fill your fridge with salmon, eggs, beef and all of that good stuff and forget about supplements.

Some people are afraid that protein supplements can cause kidney problems. The only category of people that might be in danger from a very high protein diet are people with kidney issues. This category of people is often used as a faulty generalization by mass media or other people to criticize high protein diets. Yes, protein requires more effort from your kidneys to be processed, but guess what? The kidneys are always under stress! That's what they're made for. About 20% of the blood pumped by the heart goes to the kidneys and they filter a total of 180 liters (48 gallons) of blood every single day.

Nowadays, I keep a whey protein supplement around the house and use it in the following scenarios:

a. On days that I skip a meal due to being too busy

b. On days that my diet wasn't as protein dense as I'd like it to be

c. When I want to train on an empty stomach, but I haven't had food for too many hours.

2. Creatine Monohydrate has been shown to improve power output, and is often used by athletes to increase high-intensity exercise capacity and lean body mass. It is one of the most studied supplements and it has been proven to aid muscle building goals very effectively. There is no evidence that it causes any health issues whatsoever. Keep in mind however, that there are a fair number of people who are non-responders.

Therefore, there is a possibility that you won't see any results by adding this supplement. Oh, I also forgot to mention that it's also super cheap.

My Secret Supplement

This is another substance I forgot to mention, that also has been proven to be effective. I use a caffeine supplement as a pre- and intra-workout supplement most of the days I train. It's inexpensive, you can easily find it at the supermarket, and it's called - Coffee! You add a teaspoon of it in hot water, stir and drink. I prefer ice coffee during the warm months of the year and hot coffee when it's cold.

"Doesn't Coffee Dehydrate You?" That another question I've gotten in the past and it's just another myth. Coffee, like any drink, can contribute to your daily fluid requirement. Taking that into consideration, it's mild diuretic effect doesn't have a negative effect to your total fluid volume requirements. Of course, anything in excess is not good for you, not even plain water! So, avoid extreme coffee consumption as well. Personally, I like to have on average two cups per day, and never go above three. More than that can potentially irritate your stomach and increase stress levels.

Final thoughts on supplements

As you can see my experience with supplements is quite limited, but I considered it important to mention them since this is a topic that many people frequently ask questions about. The three supplements above are the only few that are backed up by serious scientific research. If you want to supplement your athletic diet it's up to you. Make sure you choose a quality manufacturer for starters. Next, to be on the safe side, ask a nutritionist for some extra guidelines referring to dosage and any implications they might have with your other dietary habits and/or medications.

My advice is to find the weak links in your lifestyle and diet, and if you cannot fix them naturally, ask a specialist for advice on how to address these needs. Don't forget however, supplements are not magical and won't make a difference if you don't train hard enough. As a matter of fact, a no-supplement diet with a good training program will give you better results, than an average training program combined with the finest powder and pill supplements.

Don't obsess over supplements. I find that a lot of people do so which distracts them from what really delivers results – hard work.

Final thoughts on dieting advice

If you're following all the nutritional tips above, you're training hard and your weight gain or weight loss goals is still at a halt, certain health conditions should be taken into consideration. Consulting your doctor, to make sure you don't have any underlying health conditions you aren't aware of, is a good call at this point. Also, keep in mind that all the recommendations above are just suggestions, and everybody's needs differ.

Some people need more carbs to function well, while others can function better when keeping them to a minimum. Also, getting professional help if your diet is constantly failing you, is a better solution than moving from diet to diet to diet by yourself. Lastly, minors should always ask parental permission to follow a diet plan.

PART 3
EXERCISE SELECTION &
PROPER EXECUTION

Most traditional bodybuilding approaches try to isolate muscle groups and train them separately. A friend of mine call this Frankenstein training, because instead of seeing your body as an interconnected whole you try to break it down to parts. For those who like the bodybuilder physique, and training with machines/weights, it's an approach that can work. I'm assuming that this isn't why you're reading this book. Trying to structure your workouts based on muscle group isolation is a typical mistake that isn't efficient, nor does it fit the bodyweight training philosophy that we talked about in Part 1.

As we mentioned previously in the book, focusing on getting as strong as possible at the basic movement patterns (MPs) and the most efficient exercises related to these MPs, is the way to go and the secret to sculpting a calisthenics physique. To refresh our memory, let's have a look at these again:

a) Pull movements (i.e. Pull-ups and inverted rows).
b) Push movements (i.e. Pike or Handstand push-ups, regular push-ups and dips)
c) Lower-body multijointed-movements (i.e. Squatting, Lunging, vertical jumping, high intensity uphill running and stair climbing)
d) Movement (or resistance of movement) generated by the Core (i.e. Planks, leg raises, hollow body, and more.)

Keep in mind that bodyweight exercises activate a lot of muscle groups. For example, even Chin-ups have been shown in an **EMG study** to activate the chest up to 57% (!). Therefore, when I mention muscle groups activated by MPs below, keep in mind that those are simply the muscle groups that play the biggest role for each MP. At the end of the week, total training volume per muscle group balances out and your whole body is targeted. Each body part of a calisthenics physique is always the result of the combination of the following movements – not a result of any sort of isolation exercise.

Note: Keep in mind that this book is not meant to be a detailed exercise demonstration guide. You can find decent tutorials on how to execute bodyweight exercises all over the internet. But, there **are** some key technical points I want you to keep in mind with each exercise that oftentimes are not mentioned in online tutorials or demonstration books. These are the key points that I've mostly focused **on below.**

1. PULL (BACK, BICEPS AND FOREARMS)

Pulling exercises focus on the Back, Biceps and forearms. A wide, strong and carved back is part of every impressive physique and healthy body. One simply cannot look strong if he or she has a narrow, soft back. Something to keep in mind here is that building an impressive back is also a matter of muscular shoulders. Strong shoulders give more width to the upper part of the back, enhancing that V-shape we aim for in the upper body.

I think that building strong and muscular arms is a main reason most of us men got interested in strength training growing up. It's probably the primary reason we tried doing our first pull-ups and push-ups. There's simply something manly behind a pair of strong arms that every boy aspires to developing. Muscular biceps and triceps, and vascular and marble-hard forearms are part of a calisthenics physique. Combining the pushing and pulling exercises mentioned below, is key for developing them.

There are two important angles to work on when it comes to pulling if you want to build a balanced calisthenics physique – the Vertical pull and the Horizontal pull. The best exercises to target these angles are Pull-ups and Inverted rows. Later on as you advance, adding a decline pull will also add some extra volume in your upper traps – the muscles between your shoulders and neck. Upper traps are like the icing on the cake of an impressive calisthenics physique. The best exercise for them are decline inverted rows.

PULL-UPS (VERTICAL PULL)
Pull-ups are the king of all upper body exercises. Most gym rats would envy the sculpted backs of top-level gymnasts and canoe kayakers. Being a canoe kayaker in my early twenties, I know from personal experience that 95% of all top athletes in this sport do a massive number of pull-ups every week. Elite organizations such as army special forces, SWAT teams and the marines, all require a minimum number of pull-ups as a prerequisite for anyone to be allowed in their training programs. That's no coincidence...

There is no better exercise to determine one's relative and functional upper-body strength! Unfortunately, a large percentage of the general population is unable to perform a proper pull-up (probably not even if it were to save their own lives). If you're a human being, your shoulders, arms and whole body is designed to brachiate. It's just how our anatomy has been forged through hundreds of thousands of years in order to survive and thrive. Originally, most of our back muscles were involved in making our remote ancestors walk on all fours - pulling on the ground with their forelegs (arms) in order to propel themselves forward.

Once we transitioned to an upright walking style, these muscles became specialized in vertical movement, such as tree climbing. Unfortunately, we've reached a day and age where these muscles are left to weaken and atrophy as we spend a large amount of our days in a seated office lifestyle.

(Intro from my book How to Sculpt a Gymnast's Back with Pull-ups)

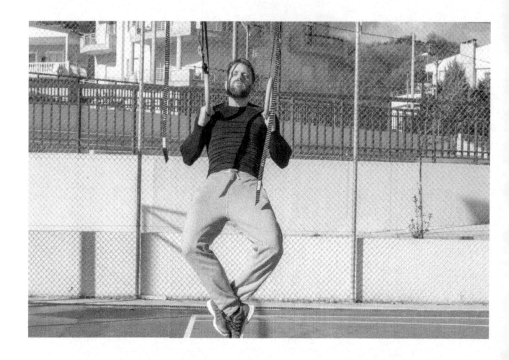

Pull-ups: The best way to determine one's relative and functional upper-body pulling strength!

Progressions for beginners

For those that find this exercise extremely challenging, the best way to get your first pull-up is working on band-assisted pull-ups in combination with inverted rows.

Assisted band pull-ups: To do assisted pull-ups grab one end of the band, throw it over the bar and pull one end through the other end to form a loop around the bar. Step one foot into the lower part of the band and wrap your other leg around the band and your shin, so it doesn't come loose as you perform your pull-ups. Find a band that has enough resistance to allow you to do six to eight reps. When you feel that you can do eight reps across all your sets easily, move to a band with two thirds or half the resistance of the initial one. Once you start feeling strong enough, start trying out normal pull-ups during every workout. At some point you'll get your first rep. After that, more reps will come a lot easier. Once you can do five normal pull-ups by bringing yourself at least eye-level parallel to the bar, stop using the bands.

If you can't afford resistance bands right now, work on the following steps...

Step #1: Passive to active hang

Hang from the pull-up bar and perform passive-to-active hang reps. A passive-hang (aka dead-hang) is when you're simply hanging off the pull-up bar, and the only muscle tension involved is that of your hands gripping the bar hard enough for you to hang. Next depress and retract your shoulder blades. This will elevate you a bit without having to bend your elbows. I also call these straight elbow pull-ups. Try to do at least five of these reps, and as you get stronger progress to ten reps. This will also train your grip if it's weak, and your upper back muscles as they will be contracting (isometrically). Once you master these techniques, combine them with the following progression.

Step #2: Negatives

a) Place a steady chair or something else that can support your weight under the pull-up bar. It should be tall enough to allow you to grab the bar at above chin level. Get on the chair/object and grip the bar. Keeping the bar at chin height, try to lower your body slowly (counting around 2-3 seconds) without depending on the chair/object. Once you lower yourself down, use the chair again to grab the bar at chin height and repeat. Depending on how easy the exercise is for you, perform 5-12 negative repetitions, with one minute rest between each set. Once you can perform 12 repetitions move onto the next progression

b) Place the chair a bit behind the pull-up bar, put one leg on the chair and pull yourself up using your leg as little as possible. Once you reach the top, remove your leg from the chair carefully and lower your body down slowly (counting 2-3 seconds). Start again with 5-12 reps and once you can perform twelve repetitions with one minute rest, move on the next phase.

c) At this point, you should be able to do at least 2-3 normal pull-ups. Begin the set by doing as many normal pull-ups as you can. Next continue with assisted pulls until you complete a total of at least 5 reps. Be patient, progress can be slow at first. Then, out of the blue you'll notice sudden progress. Eventually you'll be able to do your first pull-up. After that, before you know it you'll be doing sets of five reps and more.

Advanced Variations

Chest Height Pull-ups: These are my favorite pull-ups. They are just like normal pull-ups, but instead of raising your body until eye level with the bar, this time you will raise your body until the bar touches the height of your upper chest - just below your collarbone. This technique also maximized focus on your lats. This is because the lats are fully contracted when your shoulder are drawn down and back. Once you can perform 12-15 reps, move onto the next variation. Later on, you can go even lower, bringing the bar to the sternum.

Pull-ups With Legs Raised: This progression combines a pull and an abdominal exercise both into one because raising your legs gives your abs a great work out. Start with bended knees at 90 degrees in front of you. As this becomes easier, extend your legs until they are parallel to the floor. Once you can perform 15 reps, move onto the next variation. This is a handy variation if you're short on time and want to combine two exercises into one. If time isn't an issue, I prefer focusing on the previous variation and training your abs with other core specific exercises.

INVERTED ROWS (HORIZONTAL PULL)

The horizontal pull is as a functional movement pattern that bodyweight exercise enthusiasts quite often neglect. The best bodyweight exercise to incorporate this movement to your routine are inverted rows. Inverted rows are generally one of those exercises that just don't get enough credit. They might not be as cool as Pull-ups, but they are an amazing exercise with a ton of benefits... I'm going to blab a bit more about it in this section, hoping that you'll take it under serious consideration in your workout plan.

In order to build a strong, sculpted and symmetrical back you need the right amount of both horizontal and vertical pulling strength. Inverted rows focus more on the upper half of your back, specifically the muscles between your shoulder blades. They also contribute to the back portion of the shoulder (posterior delts). Inverted rows are considered more of a beginner's exercise, but if you practice them with perfect technique and work your way up to more advanced variations – they can serve your muscle-building goals even as an advanced trainee.

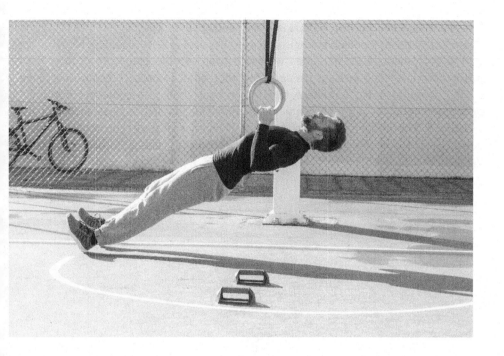

Don't neglect horizontal pulling!

The importance of balancing vertical and horizontal pull
Neglecting horizontal pulling strength and over-developing vertical pulling strength can lead to imbalances. I see this often with calisthenics enthusiasts. A lot of these guys might have incredible pull-up strength, but they often completely ignore horizontal pulling strength. A big imbalance between vertical pulling strength and horizontal pulling strength can intensify rounding of the shoulders and hyperextension in the lower back. This is due to over-development of muscles such as your lats and under-development of muscles such as the middle trapezius. Although performing your pull-ups with perfect technique reduces this effect, adding inverted rows in your routine will ensure you avoid it completely.

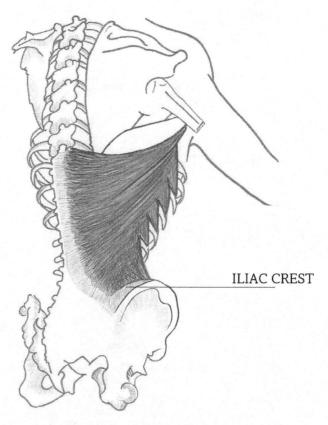

ILIAC CREST

The lats connect your arms, back and lower body all together

Inverted rows can develop scapular (shoulder-blade) stability, which promotes good posture. Strengthening and improving the function of muscles, such as the trapezius and the rhomboids (upper/middle back muscles), leads to improved scapular stabilization, which can also contribute to shoulder health. Lack and weakness of scapular function can lead to lack of stability and functionality of the shoulder. When back, shoulders and arms all work with grace and optimal synergy – your pulling strength can rise to a whole new level.

In summary: Inverted rows promote better posture and shoulder health. They contribute to overall pulling strength and play a big role in developing a functional, strong, muscular and carved back.

Decline Inverted-Rows

Place your feed on an elevated surface (i.e. bench, chair or even fit-ball). This will increase the intensity of the exercise by putting more weight on your upper body. If you want to add some extra muscle on your upper traps, increase the angle to the point that your body is at a decline level.

Full bodyweight Inverted-rows

Once you're strong enough you can progress to doing inverted rows with your feet elevated and your knees bent. Your thighs should be parallel to the floor and your knees bent at ninety degrees. You want to pull yourself up until your hands touch your lower ribs, while maintaining your elbows close to the body (don't allow them to flare out). This might be a bit difficult at first, but you'll slowly get there. The exercise is best performed on parallel dip bars or with rings. Straight bars are not that ideal since they don't allow a lot of range of motion.

One legged Inverted-row

Another good variation is to use one leg to balance your lower body while keeping the other leg extended just above the floor. This will also activate more of your core, glutes and hamstring muscles. Again, I prefer targeting the core with core-specific exercises, but if time is of essence you can hit two birds with one stone doing such variations.

Pulling Variations/Progressions to avoid

a) Wide-grip Pull-ups: Very often you'll hear people recommend wide grip pull-ups for more lat activation. In reality this variation just makes the range of motion of the exercise smaller, which actually leads to less lat activation. The main function of the lat during a pull-up is to pull the upper arm down and close to the body. When you're using a wide grip, you shorten the range of movement of that movement, and due to the angle of the arm, smaller muscles take over the stress.

Using extreme wide grips places an unnatural strain on the small muscles below your armpit (teres minor and major), increasing your possibilities for injury. I've personally strained my teres major in my early twenties from doing too many wide grip pull-ups. The tear took quite a while to heal and I had to stay off the bar for more than 5 weeks.

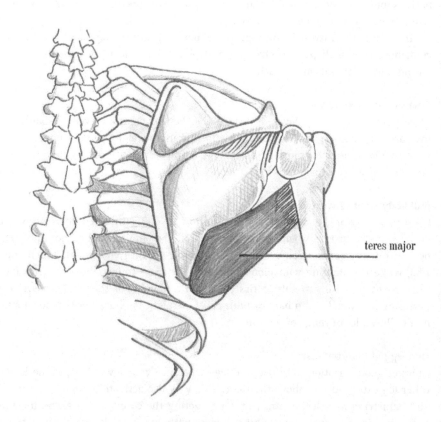

teres major

A narrower grip allows a better stretch and a more complete contraction of the lats. Both important factors for muscle growth. On the other hand, a wide grip pull-up makes it almost impossible to bring the elbows close to the body – the point where the lats are close to maximum contraction. In summary, the best grip is a normal/just-a-bit-wider-than-shoulder-width grip. This grip offers superior lat activation and low injury rate. It allows your lats to contract harder (greater muscle-fiber recruitment) at the top position of the rep and it offers a larger range of motion as you going down.

b) Chin-ups: Chin-ups and pull-ups differ mainly in the fact that they use an underhand grip. This means that your palms are facing towards you instead of facing away. I've grown less and less fond of the chin-up over the years. The first reason is that locking-out the elbows with an underhand grip places the joints of the arm in an unnatural alignment that generates excessive torsion . In other words, straightening your elbows during chin ups causes twisting forces on your wrists, elbows and shoulders. This can cause strains and issues like elbow tendonitis. The pull-up allows a more joint friendly position, greater range of motion and greater muscle activation. If you do choose to do include chin-ups in your workout routine, make sure you don't lock out (straighten) your elbow joints completely in the lower phase. Instead, keep them slightly bent. Chin-ups also serve as an easier progression for pull-ups, since some people find doing a chin-up easier than doing a pull-up.

2. PUSH (CHEST, SHOULDERS, TRICEPS)

Pushing exercises typically focus on the Chest, Shoulders and triceps. There are three main pushing MPs that help build an impressive and balanced physique. These are the horizontal push, the decline push and the incline push. Combined together they can develop impressive triceps, shoulders and a wide, rugged and pumped chest.

Other than dips, pushing exercises are the most flexible bodyweight exercises, since they require no equipment at all and they can be done anywhere. A lot of times when I'll be traveling or not in the mood to set up my gymnastic rings and do a lot of stuff, I'll just set a number of push-ups (I like to aim for 200 if it's the only thing I do that day) and that will be my workout. Sure, it's not the most balanced training approach (training full-body is always the best routine structure) but if it's just for rare occasions it's a great workout. Give it a try next time you're spending a long day at the office or trapped in an airport.

Later on, once you reach a more advanced relative strength level, you can start training the vertical pushing pattern. The best exercise here is the Handstand push-up. This is an exercise that will take your shoulder aesthetics to the next level.

PUSH-UPS (HORIZONTAL PUSH)
Push-ups... the manliest and most foundational strength exercise for the upper body. They've been turning boys into men since the dawn of physical fitness. One of the most classic bodyweight exercises. The great thing about push-ups is that they can be done anywhere! In comparison with a bench press, the push-up also requires core stability which means your abs also get a decent amount of stimulation. For a beginner, a basic

push-up may be a great challenge since it uses approximately 65% of your total bodyweight. As relative strength improves and this resistance becomes easy, some begin to either snub this exercise as too easy. Usually this is because they're unaware that they are cheating the exercise by using bad form. Performing a set of push-ups while focusing on perfect form might have you re-evaluate your thoughts on them. Then there are also one-arm push-ups, push ups on rings and a bunch of other way to keep them challenging.

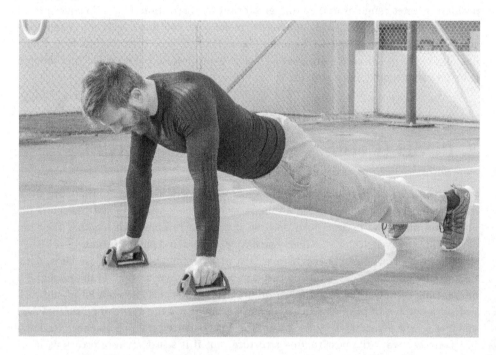

"A typical push-up requires lifting 65% of your total bodyweight"

If you have never really felt your chest working during push-ups I recommend your read my best-selling book on Amazon "How to Sculpt a Greek God Marble Chest with Push-ups".

From the book:

A few weeks ago, a guy at a calisthenics park asked me how many push-ups I can do. He was sort of polite, but his voice also had a tone of cockiness behind it. He told me he could do one hundred reps on a good day. Although physically he was quite underdeveloped (no toned chest or arms), I don't think he was lying. He actually believed he could do one hundred push-ups. But having got a glimpse of him while he was training as I entered the park, I had enough input to imagine the way he accomplished those one hundred reps. You see... doing a ton of push-ups with horrible form (i.e. using a very wide hand-stance and half the range of motion of normal push-up) can make 100 push-ups quite a feasible number for anyone that has been doing calisthenics for a while.

Now we've all seen these guys around us. Some of you probably do the same. Hey I get it, we've all been there at some point (especially as newbies). When we lack experience and proper guidance it is easy to neglect form and believe that more reps equals more gains. The truth is that the amount of unfocused reps you can do has nothing to do with how hard you're training...

Especially when aiming for gaining muscle, a proper workout should focus on muscle fatigue - not rep PRs. Intensity always trumps meaningless reps. If you want to build muscle, you should always focus on that Mind-to-muscle Connection. Don't beat up your joints and tendons with bad form and momentum. Don't use good form - use perfect form (in 9/10 of your reps at least). Be mindful, concentrated and focused. Be in the zone...

Why you need to learn how to do a one-arm push-up

Once you can do three sets of thirty perfect form push-ups, start working on one arm push-ups. Besides being an awesome exercise for triceps, chest and shoulders, it's also an amazing oblique (side ab) exercise. You might be wondering, "how in God's name are one arm push-ups going to work my side abs?". During one-arm push-ups, your obliques need to work very hard to keep the body from rotating due to the lack of stability from balancing on one arm. I still remember this... the first week I started working on one arm push-ups, I woke up the next days feeling as if someone had punched me on the side of my stomach. Sure, it's a difficult exercise and not ideal for beginners, but you can gradually build it up through the following simple progression. Start from an incline angle that allows you to do five to eight reps. Once you can do eight reps for sets, decrease the angle slowly. Using a flight of stairs to vary the angle is a good way to work on this.

PIKE PUSH-UPS (INCLINE PUSH)

Besides being a good exercise for your shoulders and upper chest, pike push-ups are a great stepping stone for preparing yourself for handstand push-ups later on. Start with basic pike push-ups. Once you can perform twelve of these, place your legs on a knee-height elevated surface and work on elevated pike push-ups until again you can perform sets of twelve reps. After that start working on the Handstand Push-up.

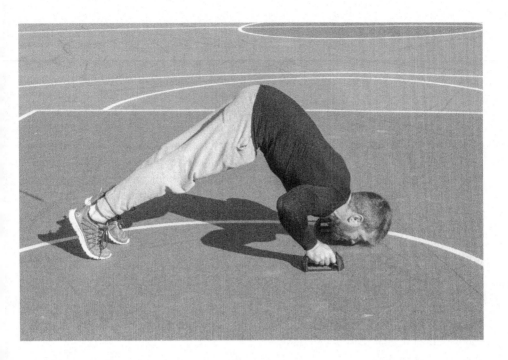

Pike push-ups

HANDSTAND PUSH-UPS (VERTICAL PUSH)

If pull-ups are the king of bodyweight training, Handstand Push-ups (HPs) are definitely the queen. Lifting your whole bodyweight in a vertical angle through your shoulders and arms is extremely challenging and the most demanding bilateral (using both limbs) bodyweight exercise of all. It requires tremendous relative upper body strength, balance and *kinaesthesia due to your body's inverted position. It is also a great exercise to strengthen the antagonistic (opposite) muscles to pull-ups. If I had to pick two exercises for developing an amazing upper physique, pull-ups and handstand push-ups would undoubtably be them. The period I started to perform handstand push-ups with good form, was one of the periods that my physique went to the next level. I gained a lot of mass in my shoulders and my body began to get that Superhero-like V-shape.

*Kinaesthesia: Awareness of the position and movement of the parts of the body by means of sensory organs (proprioceptors) in the muscles and joints.

Remember that this is a very difficult exercise. Personally, it took me 5 months of consistent training to conquer 5 reps using decent form. Start with Pike Push-ups as a progression and build it up slowly. Next use half reps (go halfway down) and then increase the range of motion gradually.

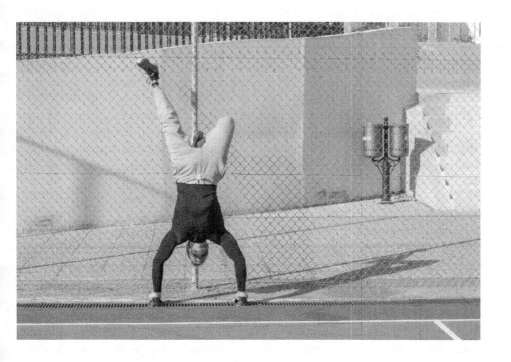

The Queen of Bodyweight Exercises

By Anthony Arvanitakis

CHEST-DIPS (DECLINE PUSH)

This is another exercise I'm going to blab a bit more about, since it is often criticized and doesn't get the credit it deserves. I think of dips as the upper-body squat. They are my favorite chest-building exercise and my favorite upper-body pushing exercise. But, one of the main reasons it catches heat is because it's thought to strain the joints and connective tissues of the shoulder. The fact that this exercise might cause problems to a lot of people doesn't mean that it's a bad exercise. Take squats for example. They are also known to cause problems to a lot of peoples' knees and lower back. If done properly though, they can be one of the best lower body exercises. The most common reason people get hurt from dips is because they don't warm up properly and/or they lack shoulder mobility. Our body is built to perform basic movement patterns that involve squatting and dipping a lot more than it's made to do bicep-curls.

Dips for shoulder health?

It's important to understand the basics of human shoulder mechanics of a pushing movement pattern such as dips. First of all, your glenohumeral joint (that's where your shoulder and upper arm connect) must be positioned properly in order to have optimal stability and produce sufficient force. Specifically, you need to start with your chest open and your shoulders pulled back and downwards (or as we'll explain in more detail later – scapular retraction and depression).

Yes, when performed incorrectly, dips can be problematic for the shoulders. But that goes for any pushing related exercise. However, when executed with perfect technique dips are actually great for shoulder health. The passive stretch you get during the lower position can increase shoulder flexibility and mobility. Most people will tell you to avoid going lower than ninety degrees of elbow flexion. This can be a good rule to keep your shoulders safe but that doesn't mean that you can't go lower if you have healthy and mobile shoulders. In reality, range of motion varies from person to person. Here's a more custom rule of thumb when it comes to personal range of motion for dips. The point you want to stop as you are lowering your body, is when you feel a light stretch in the shoulder and chest. Of course, this requires doing the exercise with complete mind-to-muscle awareness and starting off with slow tempo until you get accustomed to the technique. So, focus on perfect technical execution and move slow in the beginning.

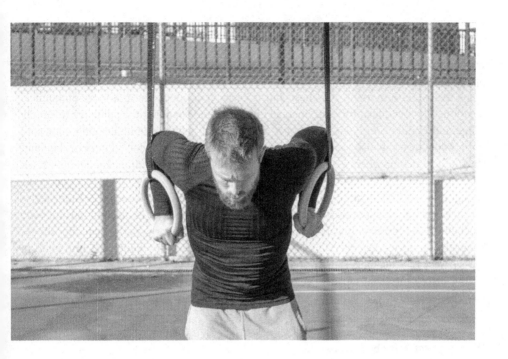

The upper-body squat...

Tips for healthy Dips

1. Learn to Hinge: Chest-dips, in comparison with straight-up dips, are performed by leaning forward (instead of standing straight) as you're performing the exercise. Specifically, you want to tilt the torso at about forty-five degrees. Not only does this focus the exercise more on the chest, but it keeps your shoulders in a more anatomical position. When you lean forward, instead of flexing and rounding the spine try to simply hinge and maintaining your spine in a more neutral position while keeping your core tight. Make sure you also keep your elbows close to the body and don't let them flare out. On the way down, when a slight stretch is felt in the chest and/or shoulders – push yourself up again.

Straight-up dips focus more on the triceps but their biggest disadvantage is that they're too stressful on the shoulders. This mainly happens because you're altering natural body mechanics and proper muscle-activation patterns. A properly performed dip should allow the stress of the exercise to be more balanced across the joints and musculature (your chest is a lot bigger than your triceps and shoulders). This means that besides saving your joints, you position your body in a position that it is stronger. This means that besides safer you are also able to do more quality reps and maximize muscle growth.

Dip progression for beginners

If dips are too challenging for you, start either with band assisted reps (google band assisted dip if you're not familiar with these) or by decreasing the range of motion if you do not have bands. Find a band-resistance or range of motion challenging enough to allow you five repetitions with clean form. Depending on which method you use, switch to a lighter band or increase the range of motion as you get stronger.

Advanced Variations – Ring dips

Ring dips force you to contract your muscles harder and recruit your stabilizing muscles. This takes the exercise to a whole new level. Shoulders, chest, arms and abs have to be constantly activated for you to maintain proper form. Unlike a dip station, the rings will sway back and forth the moment you lose focus on technique and muscle activation. You can't just jump on the rings and let your mind wander as you pump out reps. This is why I also consider them a great tool for practicing mind-muscle connection (MMC).

Because the rings want to drift outward, your chest has to be always tight to maintain them aligned. This way you get broader and deeper activation of the pectoral muscle fibers. If you're doing them for the first time and your arms are shaking like leaves, don't worry – it's normal. It takes some time getting used to them. Start slowly, simply trying to balance on the rings with your elbows straight. Gradually add some reps with limited range of motion (ROM). As you get stronger increase the ROM more and more.

MOVEMENT (OR RESISTANCE OF MOVEMENT) GENERATED BY THE CORE

The core gets plenty of activation during most bodyweight exercises. Because of that, training your core through one or two exercises twice per week can be enough. For example, do leg raises on Monday and Thursday and hollow-body on Tuesday and Friday. Focusing on getting the whole body stronger as you get leaner is the best thing to do if you want a good looking defined flat stomach. If there is one secret when it comes to impressive abs than that's it! A lean V-Shaped body will emphasize your abs way more than doing multiple mediocre core exercises. The biggest mistake you can do when trying to build impressive abs is wasting too much time obsessing on core training in expense of neglecting overall strength and multijoint exercises. This is why in this book, I'll be recommending just a few exercises that I consider the most effective for core aesthetics, functionality and health.

HOLLOW BODY HOLD
The most important thing in this exercise is to be conscious of what is happening between your upper back and the hips. You don't just want your lower back flat against the floor, you want your lower back to be applying pressure on the floor. Start with your feet and arms pointing towards the ceiling. Your extremities simply serve in increasing the intensity of the exercise. As you improve, your goal is to reach a full hollow body position without decreasing the maximum pressure your lower back can apply to the ground. The full hollow body requires holding your arms and legs extended close to parallel to the floor. Toes and fingers pointing towards the opposite direction and hands and ankle are slightly above the ground. Extended hollow body holds require high-level core strength that few people have.

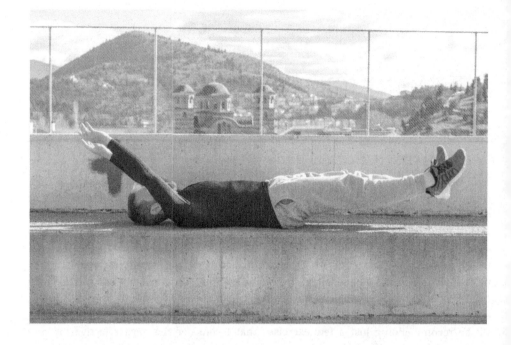

Keep the lower back flat on the ground at all times

If keeping your lower back pressing against the floor is too difficult in the beginning , you can fold your mat in a way that brings the lower back an inch or two closer to the floor. This is also a good tip for people with lordosis. Another thing to keep in your mind here is head position. Most people teach you to lift your head off the ground while doing this exercise. I prefer to allow the head to rest on the floor. The main reasons I teach the exercise this way is because it's a lot friendlier to the cervical portion of the spine and it allows you to focus on core activation. Remember, the only thing you don't want to be hollow during this exercise is your lower back and the floor beneath it.

WOODCHOPPERS

Most of us work a lot on the same basic movement patterns: Pushing and pulling horizontally (i.e push-ups and inverted rows), pushing and pulling vertically (pull-ups and handstand push-ups or pikes) and some form of squatting. Therefore, an important movement that gets commonly ignored is rotational movement. If you've been training for more than a year consistently and you've mastered basic abdominal exercises, this is an important movement you should consider incorporating into your program.

Woodchoppers are typically done at the gym with cables or dumbbells. If you train at home and you have dumbbells laying around (preferably a padded one) you can use that. If you train outdoors, an easy solution is finding a rock you can easily grip and that weights about two to three kilos (four to six pounds).

You can also do a variation of these with suspension trainers or even gymnastic rings – the standing oblique twist.

PRONE COBRA (LOWER BACK)

This is a great exercise, especially for people with a type of rounded posture, who sit at desks all day and generally have a sedentary lifestyle. If you tend to have a hyperlordotic posture, squeeze your glutes during this exercise. This will reduce over-recruitment of your low back muscles which, in this case, are probably already too stressed. Use prolonged sets of twenty to sixty seconds, with fifteen second rest periods. Start with 1-3 sets and progress until you can perform 3 sets of 60 seconds.

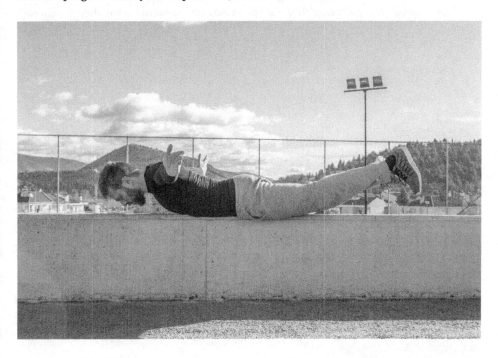

ANGELS OF DEATH (ADVANCED VARIATION)

I know, a bit of a dark name, but I found this one from Strength coach and physical therapist Jeff Cavaliere (look on Youtube for Athlean-X, a really cool channel). The Angel of death is basically a progression of the Prone Cobra. Since I hadn't seen this exercise elsewhere, I thought I'd maintain the name and give props to Jeff. From the same position as a prone cobra, bring your hands straight in front of your head with your palms rotating downwards and facing the floor. From there, bring them all the way to the back, above your glutes, with your palms rotating upwards until they touch each other.

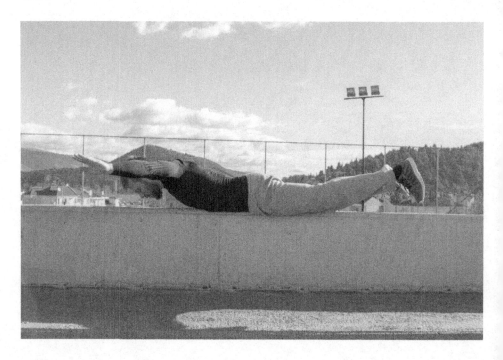

LOWER BODY TRAINING

During my journey of building muscle with bodyweight exercise, lower-body training was one of the topics that puzzled me the most. When it came to the upper body, I found that there were enough challenging exercises you can take advantage to grow stronger and bigger. But for the lower body, even though there are again a variety typical exercises to do (i.e. bodyweight squats, lunges, Skater Squats, Bulgarian squats, Shrimp squats, etc.), I found that none of these added any significant muscle mass to the lower body once you move passed your beginner gains. Sure, you can add extra weight such as sand-bags (as I've done in the past) and make these exercises more challenging. The only problem then is that you're not really doing bodyweight exercises anymore. Keeping your training routine as equipment-free as possible... Giving yourself the freedom to pack a simple backpack and train almost anywhere and anytime... these are things I like keep at the core philosophy of this book and my project – bodyweightmuscle.com.

What about pistol squats?
Some will say that you can also do pistol squats, since they're often promoted as the ultimate bodyweight exercise for training legs. I have to be honest though and tell you that I'm not a big fan of this particular exercise anymore, for a couple of reasons. For example, unless you have extreme ankle mobility it's very difficult to perform a pistol without rounding your back (lumbar flexion). Several misalignments occur in the ankle and knee joint as well (i.e. excessive pronation and valgus collapse). All these often can cause or increase knee and back pain, especially for people that are prone to such issues. I'm not saying that the pistol should be forbidden for everyone. But if you have knee and back issues, I recommend you avoid it.

Why typical bodyweight exercises won't add mass to your legs
As I kept on looking for different solutions to train my legs using strictly my own bodyweight, I came to the following simple conclusion... Your lower body is way stronger than your upper body. Therefore, it requires a lot more intensity/weight compared to what most lower bodyweight exercises can offer in order to be stimulated enough to grow stronger and bigger. So, I kept looking for extra ways to train legs. I went back to the basics, did some anatomy and biomechanics studying. Did you know, for example, that your glutes are the single biggest muscle in the human body? They help keep the torso erect and combined with the rest of your lower body muscles, they can exert the biggest force in the human body. Their main functional purpose is to allow you to jump higher and run faster.

> "Your lower body's main functional purpose is to allow you to jump higher and run faster..."

Something we forget when it comes to building muscle is that fast-twitch muscle fibers are not just stimulated when doing strength-oriented exercises. They are also recruited during high intensity anaerobic efforts and explosive movements such as plyometrics (jumping related exercises). Reminding this to myself, I realized that the best way to stimulate your legs for muscle growth, using strictly bodyweight-exercise training, doesn't require anything that complicated. You just have to train them to perform the way they were meant to perform – running fast and jumping high!

BUILDING LOWER BODY MUSCLE WITH PLYOMETRICS
During plyometrics your muscles are forced to maximize eccentric contraction (this is when the muscles contract while lengthening in simple words). An example of this is when you're landing from a jump and you want to slow down the fall. During this braking, your muscles also store elastic energy, kind of like stretching a slingshot. During a plyometric exercise, you want to quickly jump up again in order to take advantage of this elastic energy. The faster this transition, the less loss of elastic energy, and the more power output there is. Training your neuromuscular system to exploit this elastic "rebound" leads to more explosive movement, and greater recruitment of fast-twitch muscle-fibers. All this fatigue, metabolic stress and recruitment of fast twitch muscle fibers can successfully trigger muscle-growth.

In simple words... plyometrics force your muscles become more explosive and produce close-to-maximum force in short intervals of time. Simple bodyweight exercises can be turned into plyometrics by adding a simple jump between each rep. For example, squats can become jump-squats and lunges can become jumping-lunges (or plyo-lungees as I call them below).

1# PLYO-BURPEES
Plyo-burpees are a personal variation I use to target the lower body more when training legs, since regular burpees are more of a cardiovascular than a muscle-building exercise. There are two main difference between a plyo-burpee and a regular burpee. For starters, although you get into a push-up starting position, you don't actually do a push-up. Instead, you skip that part and continue the rest of the exercise by jumping forward again. Secondly, during plyo-burpees, all of your effort is focused on that last vertical jump, where you want to go as high as possible instead of just lifting your feet off the ground.

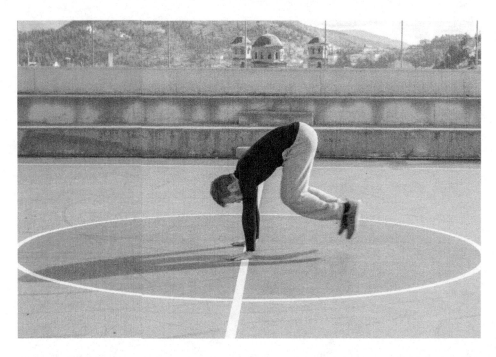

Don't just lift your feet off the ground – focus all of your effort on jumping as high as possible!

To do this efficiently, remember that as you're bringing your legs to the front from a push-up starting position into a squatted position, you're loading your muscles with elastic energy. It is this energy that has to be released quickly by jumping explosively upwards. Lastly, instead of raising your arms up during the jump (as done usually in a classic burpee), pull them backwards. I find that this allows you to focus more of the effort on your legs instead of using your arms' momentum, plus it also makes your landing smoother. To summarize everything:

a) Place your hands on the floor and kick your feet back into a push-up starting position
b) From there bring your legs forward into a squatting position (skip the push-up part)
c) Take advantage of the elastic energy that builds up when your feet land on the ground and quickly
jump high in vertical line pulling your arms backwards.
d) Land smoothly on your feet and repeat

Do 3-5 sets, starting with 6-8 reps for beginners and going up to 12-20 reps as you advance.

#2 JUMPING LUNGES

Just like in a normal lunge, take a step forward. Start the exercise by pushing off at the bottom with both feet, but focusing more on the foot in front. Switch the position of your feet during the jump and land again in a basic lunge, with the opposite leg in front this time. Try to maintain your back leg bent directly underneath your body and your front leg bent at 90 degrees at the knee and hip. Do three sets, starting with 6-8 reps as a beginner, and build it up to 30 as you advance. Including each of these exercises at least two times in your weekly routine. Combining routines like these with hill-sprints is the way to build strong, athletic and muscular legs with calisthenics.

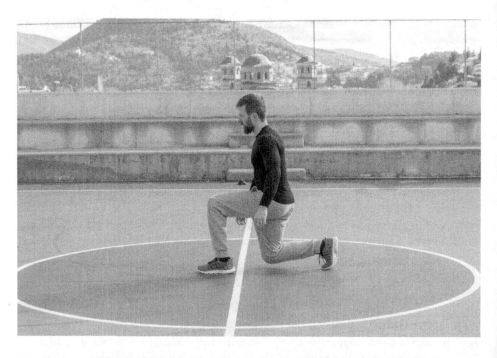

Focus on balance and keeping an upright and symmetric posture!

To watch a video tutorial of both jumping lunges and plyo-burpees, search for my channel on YouTube and look for a video called Bodyweight Plyometrics for Muscular & Defined Legs (Lower-body Calisthenics - Part 2)

Final thoughts on plyometrics
There are a few key points here to remember in order to avoid injury with plyometric exercises:

a) Introduce these gradually to your workout – start with a small jump that allows you to do six good-form reps.

b) Don't combine plyometrics with just any lower body exercise. I find that burpees and lunges are two of the best and safest exercises to do this. Avoid extreme exercises that might be too stressful on your knees and ankles.

c) Perform plyo-bodyweight exercise combos on soft surfaces (i.e. dirt or grass) where the impact from the jumps is decreased.

BUILDING LOWER BODY MUSCLE WITH UPHILL & UPSTAIRS SPRINTS

In anaerobic exercises such as sprints, your legs are forced to work for a short timespan at an intensity high enough to bring your lower-body close to momentary muscle failure. This causes your body to recruit fast-twitch fibers, which results in muscular adaptations similar to those obtained from lifting heavy weights. Using sprints strategically in your weekly routine can build strong, defined and muscular legs. In fact, they are a lot more efficient than most typical bodyweight exercises. The main issue to consider when combining HIIT (High Intensity Interval Training) with bodyweight exercises in one workout, is energy supply. Because of the high energy drainage that HIIT causes, I recommend that you avoid training in a fasted state. This can cause a lack of energy and possible muscle breakdown.

There are three reasons I prefer sprinting uphill or upstairs over flat surfaces:

1. It produces faster fast-twitch muscle fiber recruitment due to the higher energy output required
2. Uphill and upstairs running biomechanics (such as the need for more knee flexion) develop more athletic and muscular legs

3. Due to the reduced impact (your feet land more softly on the ground) there is less friction and injury potential.

Other considerations and benefits
Bodyweight exercises are usually thought of as exercises done in one static spot with a specific rep-range. To do uphill or stair sprints you need a proper location, which might be considered problematic at first for some people used to training at home or in more limited spaces. Once you find your ideal spot though, they are super easy to implement in your training routine. If you look around in most neighborhoods, you'll realize that a short warm-up jog can get you close to an ideal flight of stairs or hill you can run on. I highly recommend including at least one of these two exercises in your weekly routine. The overall benefits they offer are great – not only for building aesthetic legs, but also for overall physical and mental health. For example, they are one of the best exercises for improving your mood due to the high release of endorphins. They also are also great for bone health since they increase lower body bone density.

Training recommendations
If it's been a long time since you last ran, start with some short jogging sessions before doing high intensity running. Try jogging for fifteen to twenty minutes, two or three times a week. After a week, give high intensity running at try. Start with three sets as a beginner and build them up to six sets gradually over time. Run for thirty seconds per set and rest two to three minutes in between by walking slowly back to your starting point. Again, MMF (Momentary Muscle Failure) is key here. Don't gas out on your first set – instead find a rhythm that will allow you to run all of your sets at about the same speed. Also, make sure you do 5-7 minutes of jogging and two easy sets (50-60% intensity) before you start your fast ones. As always, proper warm up is essential.

SPECIALIZED TRAINING TECHNIQUES (STTS)

The last century as bodybuilding became popular, a variety of specialized training techniques (STTs) have been used to stimulate more muscle growth. STTs are an especially handy tool for hypertrophy-oriented bodyweight training routines when it comes to intermediate and advanced trainees. Supersets, circuit-training and rest-pause sets are some of the most popular ones. These are also the ones that are most suitable to calisthenics. They increase fatigue by pairing exercises together, reducing rest between sets or increasing repetition volume and intensity.

Mastering technique by focusing on one exercise at a time with adequate resting periods, is important when you're getting started. You don't need extreme workout plans to build muscle during your first two months of training. That's the beauty of beginner gains – even very simple, basic stuff is enough to help you grow. But after a while, your muscles become more and more desensitized to growth. You can't avoid this. Whatever you do, your body always finds a way to adapt and learn how to handle stress as efficiently as possible. It will find a way to minimize muscle cell damage and spend as little energy as possible. If your muscles could talk, after doing the same routine for a couple of months, they'd be telling you something like this: *"Look, you've been trying to trick me for a while but I now know what you're up to each time we train... I've figured out your routine and I'm not afraid by it anymore"*.

For intermediate and advanced trainees, it's important to be aware that overusing these STTs can lead to a taxing effect on the neuromuscular system that is likely to exceed its capacity for adaptation. This is why when training with STTs on a weekly basis, it's a good idea to intersperse your training with deload weeks and maintenance periods.

Supersets

Supersets (also known as paired sets) can be defined as two exercises performed in a row without any rest. Although doing paired sets gets you through the workout quicker (about half the time), research has shown us that this doesn't decrease your training volume or power output. The best way to combine exercises in a superset is by choosing exercises that share an agonist/antagonist relationship. One excellent combination are

Pull and Push exercises. This is also called agonist-antagonist paired set (APS) training. Here's the coolest thing with APS training: Not only does combining exercises this way not decrease performance, but research has shown that it can actually increase your power output in the second superset. This greater mechanical tension generated by the agonist (primary muscle) is one of the reasons superset training increases in muscular growth.

In summary: Executing two exercises consecutively increases muscular fatigue and metabolic stress, due to the reduced rest between sets. All this happens without decreasing training volume and intensity (on the contrary it can increase it), and it's a great way to trigger muscle growth.

Superset Example: Lets say you want to super-set dips and Pullups. Start off by doing one set of dips, and the moment you're done, walk straight up to your pull-up bar or set of rings and do a set of Pull-ups. That's it! Once you're done with your set of pull-ups, you've completed one superset. Rest for about two to three minutes, and then follow up with your next superset. Reps might vary a bit in the beginning until you get used to this, so don't worry if your numbers are a bit off the first week. As with all your training, find a number of reps that allows you to work close to MMF (Momentary Muscle Failure) and build that up through time.

Circuits

Circuit training is one of the best routines when it comes to combining fat-burning and muscle growth. Not only does circuit training have one of the highest energy expenditures per minute per workout, but it also keeps burning fat way after you're done training. This is because of its effect on the magnitude and duration of EPOC in comparison with traditional forms of strength training. EPOC is the Excess Post-exercise Oxygen Consumption that occurs after an intense workout. Your body has to work extra hard to restore all your systems (things such as bod-temperature, heart rate, blood pressure, etc.), or as it is called more scientifically – homeostasis. So, even though your workout is over, your body continues to burn plenty of calories for hours after that.

Circuits also spike feel-good hormones (i.e. endorphins) a decent spike and produce a great post-workout muscle pump (good time to take a selfie?!). Plus, they allow you to perform a lot of exercises in a short amount of time. This means you get a lot done, in terms of training-volume and high intensity, in a small amount of little time. Just like with supersets, they're quite handy for busy individuals.

The best way to structure a circuit is to set up a series of exercise stations that alter the main targeted muscle groups. This is important for performance and in order to stimulate that agonist-antagonist effect we talked about in Supersets. For example, try to alternate between pull, push, lower body and core-oriented exercises. Move from one exercise to the next with minimal rest (try to keep the transition lower than 15 seconds). Ideally start with the most difficult exercises. A muscle-building oriented circuit set can have anywhere between four to six exercises. Start with three sets, and if you want to make things more challenging, add a fourth one set after six weeks.

Rest Pause Sets

The Rest/Pause technique was popularized by a famous 1960's power-lifter named Jim Williams. In his early life, big Jim had been involved in some criminal activity and was sentenced to ten years in prison. Jim turned his jail sentence into an opportunity to transform himself into the prison's strongest inmate. Although I don't condone criminal activity, I definitely like Jim's mentality on taking advantage of a bad situation and making something out of it. Later on, he also broke world bench-press records, being the first man in history to bench press 300 kg (661.41 bs) in competition. Due to the limited equipment available in the prison, Jim developed rest pause sets to help him train hard without using a lot of weight. This training method not only helps fatigue the muscle fibers but it can also help you break through challenging strength and muscle-growth plateaus.

A Rest-pause set (RPS) starts with a normal set, followed by a resting period of about ten seconds, followed by a few extra reps. For example, let's say you normally do eight pull-ups in a regular set. In a rest pause set you'd be doing eight reps, followed by ten seconds of rest, followed by a few more reps. How many more reps? As many as you can, without messing up your form. The benefit of rest-pause sets is that they allow you to increase high-quality rep volume in each set. The reason I say high-quality, is because those extra reps you add, instantly stimulate a high percentage of fast-twitch muscle fiber. This is because your muscles are still stimulated and drained from the reps you did ten seconds ago.

Trisets

Another STT I didn't mention in the beginning of this Part is trisets. A triset consists of three different exercises performed one after another, without any rest in between. They're actually just like a circuit, but with less stations/exercises. I don't use these for hypertrophy purposes, but rather for deload weeks or maintenance periods. By including a pull, a push and a lower body exercise, you can get a total-body workout in fifteen to twenty minutes max. Three sets will usually do for maintenance or deload weeks.

PART 4
BODYWEIGHT PROGRAM DESIGN

Building an impressive physique...

Gaining quality muscle mass that will stick to your body...

Creating a fit lifestyle instead of... going all out for a few weeks and then quitting because you end up injured, overwhelmed or simply bored...

These are all things that require designing a quality workout plan. Such a plan has to be approached with "a marathon and not a sprint mentality". Sure, you can start hardcore from the beginning, overtrain, and see some decent results within a few weeks. But, here's what usually happens after that. Besides the fact that you'll be flirting with injury, you'll also hit a plateau pretty soon. This can be very demotivating when you're first getting started. Overtraining doesn't only take place in your body – it also takes place in your mind. This means that if you start with extremes, you'll usually end up too drained mentally to continue training at the same pace. This is the reason why most people quit after finishing a short-term, hardcore workout plan or diet. Hey, I'm guilty of this mentality multiple times in the past, and I'm not talking just about training. Somewhere around my early thirties though, I started approaching life with a more long-term and well-thought out strategy. This was when everything started changing. Training, business and personal life began to improve in a lot more stable, steady and balanced way. Sure, it took me a while but better late than never.

Patience and strategy are the best friends of success. As a beginner, the awesome thing is that if you train properly, you don't have to overdo it in order to see progress. So, don't train randomly, have a plan and take things one step at a time. Focus initially on proper technique and keeping your joints healthy. This way you'll build a solid base for long-term progress.

How long does it take to reach your ultimate potential?
By now, you should have understood that you can't reach your ultimate potential within a few weeks or months. It's a process that takes time. How much time? Well, assuming that your diet is decent and you're training smart, about 2-3 years of serious training will get you pretty close to it. Ok, right now that might not sound that motivating. But, here's the good news! You can gain more than half of those results in less than a year!

Gaining more than half of your life's muscle-potential (while also losing fat) in just one year?

I remember my first year of training for my hometown rowing team when I was thirteen. Within just a few months, I improved my racing time (a two-kilometer rowing–ergometer test) by twenty seconds. At this rate, I thought, I'll be in the national team within no time! Needless to say, that's not how things work with exercise... whether that's sport specific performance or building an aesthetic bodyweight physique. Things go fast at first, then progress gradually starts to slow down.

But what's great with fitness is that with a proper plan, you can completely change your physique within just one year of training. To give you a more visual idea of how all this happens, let's check out the geeky diagram below.

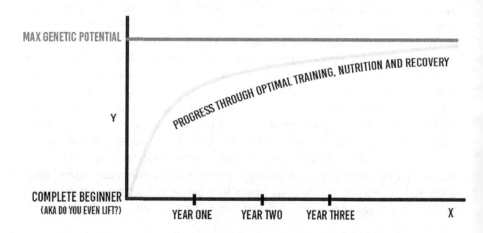

"Within the 1st year of training, you can gain up to half of the total muscle you'll be gaining during the rest of your life!"

The yellow line in the diagram, represents your progress. As you can see from the steep initial upward slope, things go pretty fast in the beginning. This only lasts for about a year though. I know, if only it continued that way...

Another cool thing that happens during your newbie training period is that you can lose fat while building muscle. Although a popular belief is that this is not possible, it actually isn't that difficult to achieve in the beginning. The only problem is that it becomes more and more difficult as you become more advanced. Still, it's very doable when you're getting started. Again, this requires a proper workout plan and a good diet to support it. Things such as making sure you're supplying your muscles with enough protein while basing your diet on healthy and minimally processed foods are essential prerequisites.

ONE-YEAR SCIENCE-BASED WORKOUT PLAN FOR BUILDING AESTHETIC BODYWEIGHT MUSCLE

Next, we'll be talking about basic principles that go into program design, in case you want to create your own plan. At the end, I'll also share with you my most successful one-year plan for building aesthetic bodyweight muscle. I've made my best gains training with this programing, and so have all of my clients who have followed it through until the end. If you're serious with your training and muscle-building goals, it's a plan I highly recommend.

There are three main ingredients that go into a successful bodyweight training plan for building muscle:
   a) Time blocks, such as Macro (weeks or months) and Micro-cycles (days or weeks)
   b) Training Load and Intensity progression from time-block to time-block (increasing sets and adding more challenging training methods)
   c) Deloading weeks and maintenance periods (training light for limited time-spans, but also taking it easier for longer periods once in a while).

Since we've covered b) and c) earlier in the book, let's have a look at time-blocks and why they're so important when designing a program or following one that uses them.

Macro and micro-cycles
Macro and micro-cycles are time units used for systematic planning of physical training. They are useful for increasing and cycling important muscle-building variables in a training program, such as intensity and training volume. They can also divide the year into different phases which focus on different goals (i.e. gaining muscle vs muscle mass maintenance). Macro and micro-cycles are the first component you need to take into consideration when setting your workout plan. Macrocycles give you more of a long-term (usually monthly) view, and Microcycles give you more of a day to day/weekly view of your workout plan.

In the plan I'll be sharing with you, each macro cycle will usually consist of six weeks, and each micro-cycle will consist of seven days. There's only one exception in the last phase of the plan, where the last macrocycle lasts three weeks. There is a reason I've organized most macrocycles in six-week periods. I've found that when it comes to getting stronger and gaining muscle with calisthenics, on average, most people experience plateaus every six weeks. Therefore, making little tweaks every six weeks help you to keep you progressing. As my favorite strength training coach and author Dan John says: *"Everything works, for about six weeks..."*

97

This doesn't mean that you have to completely change your workout plan. That would only have you running in circles. Having no reference points means you have no way to compare your progress and push yourself to improve. Instead you want to change little things and leave the core of your program intact.

Your first adjustments should include increasing training volume, based on the recommendations we discussed in the training-volume chapter. You can do that by adding more training sets per movement pattern or adding one exercise per movement pattern. Another way to make your program more challenging once you move passed your beginner phase, is to increase intensity by adding specialized training. Do this gradually, don't change every day's workout! Instead start with changing one or two workouts of the week.

i.e. if you train four days a week doing straight-sets, replace two of those straight-set days with supersets

When setting up a long-term plan, it's good to consider important future dates when training will be challenging (vacations, travelling, busy work periods, etc..). For example, for some people it's a good idea to plan times off and maintenance periods when they're on summer vacation. I like to take time off during summer holidays and do the opposite during winter holidays. Here's what I mean. I like to plan the most challenging training periods of the year during times such as Christmas holidays and New-Years Eve. During such times, I know there will be a ton of tasty food around me. Avoiding some indulgence during such times is no fun for me. I rather have those extra calories fuel a challenging workout and build more muscle than let them go to waste and turn into fat. Enjoying a rich and warm holiday meal after a cold and tough outdoor workout is one of my favorite things in life!

Right now, it's Christmas as I'm finishing this book, and I hear fitness experts sharing all kinds of advice on how to avoid overeating. What I like to say is "It's not what you do between Christmas and New Year's Eve, but what you do between New Year's Eve and Christmas that matters. So train hard and enjoy that stuffed turkey!"

How to adjust this plan to your current level
If you're a complete beginner, then definitely start this program from the beginning. I just mention this because sometimes people think that beginning at the advanced phase of a workout plan will give them advanced results. It doesn't work like that. You need to work on your foundation first! Are you someone who has done a bit of bodyweight training at some point of your life and right now you are out of shape? Again, start this program from the beginning.

For those who are truly more advanced, here's what you can do. Start by calculating your weekly training volume per movement pattern to get a good estimate of where you're at as a bodyweight trainee. Let's have a look again at the weekly volume guidelines, so you estimate where you're at.

a) Beginner: 10-12 sets per movement pattern
b) Intermediate: 12-14 sets per movement pattern
c) Advanced: 14-18 sets per movement pattern

After this, here's what I recommend next:

- Intermediate: If you're an intermediate bodyweight-exercise trainee, meaning you've been training for more than six weeks consistently and your weekly volume per movement pattern is between twelve and fourteen sets, start the following program from Phase 2: Macrocycle 1.
- Advanced: If you've been training for more than four months consistently and your weekly volume per movement pattern exceeds fourteen sets, start from Phase 2: Macrocycle 2.
- More advanced: For a more advanced trainee, I find it best that you study the whole plan and calibrate by yourself what's the best place to start.

The Plan

The following plan is what I've found to be the best way to make consistent progress when you're trying to build muscle with calisthenics. The plan starts by dividing your workout plan into three phases: A Beginner's phase, an Intermediate phase and an Advanced phase. Each phase consists of one to two Macrocycles that last six weekly microcycles each. These microcycles follow a 5:1 load to deload pattern. What does this mean? It means that every five weeks of normal training volume and intensity, you'll have one week during which you'll take things a bit easier. All this creates a wave-like loading pattern that will allow for gradual steady progress and muscle gains of course! If you do this properly, you'll take advantage of the overreaching and supercompensation principles while staying away from plateaus and overtraining.

Side-note: *Kindle books don't allow special formatting which makes it difficult for me to give you the following workout plan in a more graphic and eye-friendly structure. If you'd like an excel-sheet type of format of my workout plan, feel free to mail me at info@bodyweightmuscle.com. Make sure you use the following subject in your email: Bodyweight Muscle Sheet.*

Here's a brief overview of the plan:
Phase 1 (Beginner), Macrocycle A (6 weeks)
Phase 2 (Intermediate), Macrocycle A (6 weeks)
Phase 2 (Intermediate), Macrocycle B (6 weeks)
Phase 3 (Advanced), Macrocycle A (6 weeks)
Phase 3 (Advanced), Macrocycle B (3 weeks)

BEGINNER PHASE

Everybody's weight, height and body proportions differ. This can make some exercises more challenging for some than they are for others. Two common exercises that a lot of people struggle with in the beginning are pull-ups and/or dips. For example, for those who weigh a bit more than average and/or have longer limbs, it makes sense that they'll need more time to master pull-ups. Afterall, it is an exercise that requires lifting your whole bodyweight. It is a big difference if that bodyweight is two-hundred pounds instead of a more average weight like one-hundred and sixty pounds. If some exercises of the plan are too challenging for you, don't worry, you can still use the program. All you need to do is find an easier progression to work on. Can't do pull-ups? Work on assisted band pull-ups. Can't do inverted rows with your feet straight? Start with knees bent. Go back to the exercise selection chapter, and look for easier progressions that you can use. As you get stronger, work your way up to more difficult progressions and variations.

Here's a brief breakdown of the Beginner's phase Macrocycle...

Microcycle 1: Introduction (Workout A)
Microcycle 2: Introduction (Workout A)
Microcycle 3: Add more exercises and change the workout frequency (Workout A & B)
Microcycle 4: Repeat week 3
Microcycle 5: Repeat week 3
Microcycle 6: Deload week

MICROCYCLES 1,2 (ADAPT TO BODYWEIGHT EXERCISE & BUILD CONSISTENCY & DISCIPLINE)

The first two weeks are introductory. You'll be training three times a week, which is enough frequency to stimulate muscle growth, while also allowing your body to gradually adapt to the exercises. Having a minimum of a full day of recovery between each workout is always a good idea when you're getting started. This is the workout:

Workout A: (Monday, Wednesday, Friday)
1. Pull-ups: 3 sets, 4 – 12 reps
2. Push-ups 3 sets, 4 –12 reps
3. Lunges: 3 sets, 8 – 30 reps (4-15 per leg)
4. Plank: 2 sets, 15 – 60 seconds
5. Prone Cobra: 2 sets, 15 – 60 seconds

During this initial phase, it's important to realize that besides building muscle, you're also working on incorporating a new habit into your weekly routine and lifestyle. Developing discipline and work-ethic are even more important than building muscle during these first two weeks. Once you find your rhythm, and consistency is not a problem, muscle will come as a natural side-effect.

As a matter of fact, there are plenty of positive side-effects. Once you have a fitness routine dialed into your weekly schedule – it will trigger a domino effect of more and more positive changes in your life. There's something about incorporating fitness in your lifestyle that makes other positive habits easier to apply. As Charles Duhigg says in his book - The Power of Habit: *"When you start habitually exercising, you start changing other, unrelated patterns in your lives, often unknowingly. Typically, people who exercise start eating better and becoming more productive at work. They smoke less and show more patience with colleagues and family. They use their credit cards less frequently and say they feel less stressed. It's not completely clear why. But for many people, exercise is a keystone habit that triggers widespread change."*

MICROCYCLES 3,4,5 (ADD JUMPING LUNGES, PLYO-BURPEES, INV. ROWS AND DIPS)

On week three you'll be adding one new exercise per movement pattern. Plyo-burpees (dynamic lower-body), dips (Push), and inverted rows (Pull). To handle your new increased training volume efficiently, you'll be switching to a four-day per week training frequency. This way you can focus on one pull, one push, one lower body and one core exercise on every workout.

Most of this book uses this four-day workout per week format. I find that it's also a great frequency for establishing a healthy habit in your weekly routine. That way, you train almost every working day, while also having a spare day midweek. This is a good way to get other weekday things done like going to your dentist, going to the municipality for paperwork, visiting your accountant or lawyer, etc.

Workout A (Monday, Thursday)
1. Pull-ups: 3 sets, 4-12 reps
2. Push-ups 3 sets, 4-12 reps
3. Jumping Lunges: 3 sets, 10 – 30 reps (5-15 per leg)
4. Plank: 2 sets, 15 – 60 seconds

Workout B (Tuesday, Friday)
1. Dips: 3 sets, 4 – 12 reps
2. Inverted-rows: 3 sets, 4-12 reps
3. Plyo-Burpees: 3 sets
4. Prone Cobra: 2 sets, 15 – 60 seconds

NOTE: You can of course pick different days of the week to train if that suits you. Just make sure they are in the same order.

MICROCYCLE 6 (Deload week)

Week six is a deload week. You only have two training days with limited training volume. Even if you feel like training more, I highly recommend taking it easy and allowing yourself to start next week with your mental and physical batteries replenished. As we said, building muscle is a long-term game and you'll want to maintain a healthy appetite for training. There's no reason to overdo it in the beginning.

Workout A (Tuesday)
1. Dips: 2 sets, 4 – 12 reps
2. Inverted-rows: 2 sets, 4-12 reps
3.Plyo-Burpees: 2 sets, 5 – 30 reps

Workout B (Thursday)
1. Pull-ups: 2 sets, 4 – 12 reps
2. Push-ups 2 sets, 4-12 reps
3. Plyo-burpees: 2 sets, 10 – 30 reps (5-15 per leg)

Note #1 on deload weeks: Keep in mind that the week after your deload week, you might sometimes notice a small decrease in performance during the first two days. Don't worry though, this is totally normal. This is just your body re-readjusting to the workout's volume/intensity. Remember this and don't overexert yourself, trying to replicate your performance from the week prior to the deload. By the end of the first week or beginning of the second of your new macrocycle, not only will get back on track, but you'll possibly be breaking a couple of plateaus. This is just the natural delayed rebounding effect from your deload week!

Note #2 for those struggling with consistency: If you're struggling with staying disciplined with your workouts, I highly recommend reading my other book "How To Never Skip Your Workout Again". In this book I share with you all kinds of practical mind-hacks, for staying disciplined to your training schedule. Here's a small part of it's introductory chapter:

"We all know that exercise is not just about looking good without a shirt on. Yet, that's one of our biggest motives. This isn't a bad thing, but it's good to remind ourselves that exercise is a very powerful tool that has more to offer than superficial benefits. Here are some of the major ones that you should always keep in mind:

- It's one of the best investments you can make for your physical health.
- It's also one of the best investments for your wallet. Think of how much money you save from future medical treatments you can potentially avoid, if you stay healthy most of your life.
- It's been proven to be one of the strongest tools for improving your mood (proven to be even more powerful than antidepressant drugs in some studies).
- It increases positive character traits such as self-confidence
- It can create a domino effect of positive change in the rest of the areas of your life

From my book "*How to never skip your workout again*".

INTERMEDIATE PHASE

This phase consists of two macrocycles. During these macrocycles you'll keep on challenging your neuromuscular system, by increasing training volume and intensity. Volume will increase by adding more sets and some new exercises. Intensity will increase by adding specialized training techniques such as super sets and high-intensity uphill and stair running.

MACROCYCLE A

Quick overview of this phase's first Macrocycle (A):

Microcycle/Week 1: Incorporate uphill and stair sprints twice a week, add hollow body and angel of death (new core exercises)

Microcycle 1: Add high intensity running, Hollow Body and Angel of Death

Microcycle 2: Repeat the previous week

Microcycle 3: Add Super-Sets twice a week

Microcycle 4: Repeat week 3

Microcycle 5: Repeat week 3

Microcycle 6: Deload week

Microcycles 1,2 (ADD HIGH INTENSITY RUNNING, HOLLOW BODY AND ANGEL OF DEATH)

In the past, I used to not be a big fan of starting your workout with cardiovascular related exercise. This is because I felt that it took a bit of my edge from the rest of the workout. But, I have found that high-intensity running doesn't affect my upper body performance. Give it a week to adjust and you'll see that, as long as you give your body 3-5 minutes to actively rest as you're prepping for the rest of the workout, you feel strong and even more energized during the rest of the workout.

Two more new exercises here will be the Hollow body (ab exercise) and Angels of death (lower-back exercise).

Workout A1 (Monday)

1. Pull-ups: 3 sets, 4 – 12 reps
2. Push-ups 3 sets, 4-20 reps
3. Plyo-Burpees: 3 sets, 8 – 30 reps
4. Hollow body: 2 sets, 15 – 60 seconds

Workout B1 (Tuesday)
1. Dips: 3 sets, 4 – 12 reps
2. Inverted-rows: 3 sets, 4-20 reps
3. Plyo-burpees: 3 sets, 5 – 30 reps
4. Angel of Death: 2 sets, 8-20 reps

Workout A2 (Thursday)
1. Uphill or stair sprints: 3 X 30" (2-3 minutes rest between each sprint)
   Short 3'-5' active break (set up equipment)
2. Pull-ups: 3 sets, 4-12 reps
3. Push-ups 3 sets, 4-20 reps
4. Hollow body: 2 sets, 15 – 60 seconds

Workout B2 (Friday)
1. Uphill or stair sprints: 3 X 30" (2-3 minutes rest between each sprint)
   Short 3'-5' active break (set up equipment)
2. Dips: 3 sets, 4 – 12 reps
3. Inverted-rows: 3 sets, 4-20 reps
4. Angel of Death: 2 sets, 8-20 reps

Adjustment 1 (not a fan of running?): Some people are not able to include high intensity running in their training. Either it's because they can't train outdoors, they have some injury that bothers them, or maybe it's just not their cup of tea. Whatever the case might be, if you're not able to run, you can keep on training your lower body based on the previous macrocycle's approach. Simply alternate plyo-burpees with jumping lunges. To be more specific, instead of starting workout A2 and B2 with high intensity running, skip that and add jumping lunges or plyo burpees as a third exercise (before your core exercises).

Adjustment 2 for more shoulder activation: If you want to prioritize your shoulders a bit more at this point, you can switch the regular push-ups with pike push-ups (and later on even progress to Handstand push-ups). Since chest-dips cover the horizontal/incline pushing movement pattern to a fair extent, you can add this iteration while maintaining your program balanced.

Microcycles 3,4,5 (ADD SUPERSETS AND INCREASE RUNNING VOLUME)
During these weeks you'll be adding Supersets for most of your exercises. Let's quickly summarize and remind ourselves the benefits of supersets: Supersets are great for increasing intensity and metabolic stress to challenge your body and stimulate more hypertrophy.

Workout A1 (Monday)

1. *Superset Pull-up and push-ups (3 sets)*
   a) Pull-ups: 4 – 12 reps
   b) Push-ups: 4-20 reps
2. *Superset Plyo-Burpees & hollow body (3 sets)*
   a) Plyo-Burpees: 8 – 30 reps
   b) Hollow body: 15 – 60 seconds

Workout B1 (Tuesday)

1. *Superset Dips and Inverted-rows (3 sets)*
   a) Dips: 4 – 15 reps
   b) Inverted-rows: 4-20 reps
2. *Superset Plyo-Burpees & Angel of death (3 sets)*
   a) Plyo-burpees: 5 – 30 reps
   b) *Angel of Death: 8-20 reps*

Workout A2 (Thursday)

1. Uphill or stair sprints: 4 X 30" (2-3 minutes rest between each sprint)
   Short 3'-5' break (set up equipment)
2. *Superset Pull-up and push-ups (3 sets)*
   a) Pull-ups: 4 – 12 reps
   b) Push-ups: 4-12 reps
2. Hollow body: 3 sets, 15 – 60 seconds

Workout B2 (Friday)

1. Uphill or stair sprints: 4 X 30" (2-3 minutes rest between each sprint)
   Short 3'-5' break (set up equipment)
2. *Superset Dips and Inverted-rows (3 sets)*
   a)   Dips: 4 – 15 reps
   b)   Inverted-rows: 4-12 reps
3. Angel of Death: 3 sets, 8-20 reps

Microcycle 6 (DELOAD WEEK)
As usual, week six is a deload week. You'll be giving your body complete rest from high intensity running and you'll focus on maintaining your strength. Do about 20% less reps (i.e. instead of 10 pull-ups go for eight) and if you feel like going for a run you can do a fifteen to twenty-minute jog. Stay below 140 heartbeats/minute and do it on a flat soft surface (i.e. dirt or grass). If you feel more like doing some hill-sprints or stair, go for three to four sets at 65-70% intensity.

Workout A (Tuesday)
1. Dips: 3 sets, 4 – 12 reps
2. Inverted-rows: 3 sets, 4-12 reps
3. Plyo-Burpees: 2 sets, 5 – 30 reps
4. Angel of Death: 3 sets, 8-20 reps

Workout B (Thursday)
1. Pull-ups: 3 sets, 4 – 12 reps
2. Push-ups 3 sets, 4-12 reps
3. Plyo-Burpees: 2 sets, 10 – 30 reps (5-15 per leg)
4. Plank: 2 sets, 15 – 60 seconds

MACROCYCLE B
Quick Overview of Macrocycle B
Microcycles 1,2: Repeat Week 5 from Intermediate Macrocycle A
Microcycle 3: Add circuit training twice a week
Microcycles 4,5: Repeat week 3
Microcycle/Week 6: Deload week

Microcycles 3,4,5 (ADD CIRCUIT TRAINING AND INCREASE SPRINTING SETS)
Workout A1 (Monday)
Circuit training (3 sets)
   a) Pull-ups: 4 – 12 reps
   b) Push-ups: 4-20 reps
   c) Plyo-Burpees: 8 – 30 reps
   d) Hollow body: 15 – 60 seconds

Workout B1 (Tuesday)
Circuit Training (3 sets)
   a) Dips: 4 – 15 reps
   b) Inverted-rows: 4-20 reps
   c) Plyo-burpees: 5 – 30 reps
   d) Angel of Death: 8-20 reps

Workout A2 (Thursday)
1. Uphill or stair sprints: 5 X 30" (2-3 minutes rest between each sprint)
   Short 3'-5' break (set up equipment)
2. *Superset Pull-up and push-ups (3 sets)*
   a) Pull-ups: 4 – 12 reps

   b) Push-ups: 4 - 20 reps
3. Hollow body: 15 – 60 seconds

<u>Workout B2 (Friday)</u>
1. Uphill or stair sprints: 5 X 30" (2-3 minutes rest between each sprint)
    Short 3'-5' break (set up equipment)
2. *Superset Dips and Inverted-rows (3 sets)*
  a) Dips: 4 – 15 reps
  b) Inverted-rows: 4 -20 reps
3. Angel of Death: 3 sets, 8-20 reps

Microcycle 6 (DELOAD WEEK)
Again, you'll be giving your body complete rest from high-intensity running and focus on maintaining your strength. Do about 20% less reps and if you feel like going for a run you can do a fifteen to twenty-minute jog. Stay below 140 heartbeats/minute and do it on a flat soft surface (i.e. dirt or grass). As previously, if you feel more like doing some hill-sprints or stair, go for three to four sets at 65-70% intensity.

   <u>Workout A1 (Tuesday)</u>
   Circuit training (3 sets)
  a) Pull-ups: 4 – 12 reps
  b) Push-ups: 4-20 reps
  c) Plyo-Burpees: 8 – 30 reps

   <u>Workout B1 (Thursday)</u>
   Circuit Training (3 sets)
  a) Dips: 4 – 15 reps
  b) Inverted-rows: 4-20 reps
  c) Plyo-burpees: 5 – 30 reps

ADVANCED PHASE

The advanced phase consists of two Macrocycles (A,B). During these macrocycles, you'll keep on challenging your body to build muscle by adding volume (sets) and intensity (specialized training). Your last macrocycle is the only macrocycle that is half in duration (three microcycles), but it's also quite intense. I call these weeks hell-weeks, just like the Navy SEAL's call the hardest week of their training. Hey, at least you won't have to go through a week of being stranded in the middle of the ocean at a dessert island, feeling cold and hungry, while getting less than four hours of sleep per day.

The advanced phase simply adds two more training days (you train six days in total) during your second and third week, which will be short and focused on your most challenging exercises. Therefore, once you're done with the advanced phases, I highly recommend ten to fourteen days of rest.

MACROCYCLE A

Quick overview of Macrocycle A (Advanced phase):
Microcycles/Weeks 1,2: Repeat microcycle 3 from macrocycle B of the previous phase.
Microcycle/Week 3: Increase volume
Microcycle/Week 4,5: Repeat
Microcycle/Week 6: Deload week

Microcycles 3,4,5 (Increase training volume and add side to side hollow body rocks)

Workout A1 (Monday)
Circuit training (4 sets)
  a) Pull-ups: 4 – 12 reps
  b) Push-ups: 4-20 reps
  c) Plyo-Burpees: 8 – 30 reps (15 per leg)

Workout B1 (Tuesday)
Circuit Training (4 sets)
  a) Dips: 4 – 15 reps
  b) Inverted-rows: 4-20 reps
  c) Plyo-burpees: 5 – 30 reps

Workout A2 (Thursday)
1. Uphill or stair sprints: 6 X 30" (2-3 minutes rest between each sprint)
    Short 3'-5' break (set up equipment)

2. *Superset Pull-up and push-ups (4 sets)*
   a) Pull-ups: 4 – 12 reps
   b) Push-ups: 4-20 reps
3. Side to Side Hollow body rocks: 15" – 60"

Workout B2 (Friday)
1. Uphill or stair sprints: 6 X 30" (2-3 minutes rest between each sprint)
   Short 3'-5' break (set up equipment)
2. *Superset Dips and Inverted-rows (4 sets)*
   a) Dips: 4 – 15 reps
   b) Inverted-rows: 4-20 reps
3. Side to Side Hollow body rocks: 15" – 60"

Note: At this point your training is challenging enough that your core gets a large amount of stimulation just indirectly through multijoint exercises. You'll be only focusing on one advanced variation for your abs, the Side-to-side Hollow-body-rock. Make sure you've mastered regular hollow body holds before you move to this progression. Side to side hollow body rocks also focus a bit more on your obliques (side abs).

Microcycle 6 (DELOAD WEEK)

Workout A1 (Tuesday)
Circuit training (4 sets)
   a) Pull-ups: 4 – 12 reps
   b) Push-ups: 4-20 reps
   c) Plyo-Burpees: 8 – 30 reps (15 per leg)

Workout B1 (Thursday)
Circuit Training (4 sets)
   a) Dips: 4 – 15 reps
   b) Inverted-rows: 4-20 reps
   c) Plyo-burpees: 5 – 30 reps

MACROCYCLE B
These last two weeks are not easy. But, getting through them is mostly a matter of being mentally strong. Your body naturally doesn't like being beyond its limits or even what it is currently used to. So, once you switch from a four-day training schedule to a six-day

one, it will start complaining. But, if you just switch off that inner nagging voice and take it one rep at a time, I promise you you'll make it. You'll slowly discover that "mind over matter" is not just a phrase. Relax your face as you go into the first sets of the workout. If your body says "I feel too heavy", simply smile and imagine that you're ten pounds lighter.

The more you try to buy into this belief, the more you'll be amazed by how it will affect your performance and the ease of the rest of the workout. If you're skeptic like me, right now you feel that all this is just sounds like a pseudoscientific paragraph from a book like the "The secret". What you maybe don't know though, is that there have been studies confirming that your beliefs can affect your strength. As one of these studies revealed: "significantly higher strength performances were observed when the resistance was greater than the subject believed". In other words, when the trainees were told that the weight they were lifting was lighter than how much it actually weighed, they did more repetitions!

Quick overview of Macrocycle B:
Microcycle/Week 1: Repeat last workout prior to deload week
Microcycles/Weeks 2,3: Add two more short Rest-pause workouts
Take ten to fourteen days off

Microcycles 2,3: HELL-WEEKS (Increase training frequency – add two rest-pause set workouts)

Workout A1 (Monday)
Circuit training (4 sets)
  a) Pull-ups: 4 – 12 reps
  b) Push-ups: 4-20 reps
  c) plyo-Burpees: 8 – 30 reps

Workout B1 (Tuesday)
Circuit Training (4 sets)
  a) Dips: 4 – 15 reps
  b) Inverted-rows: 4-20 reps
  c) Plyo-burpees: 5 – 30 reps

Workout A2 (Wednesday)
1. Uphill or stair sprints: 6 X 30" (2-3 minutes rest between each sprint)
   Short 3'-5' break (set up equipment)
2. *Superset Pull-up and push-ups (4 sets)*
  a) Pull-ups: 4 – 12 reps

b) Push-ups: 4-20 reps

3. Side to Side Hollow body rocks: 15" – 60"

<u>Workout B2 (Thursday)</u>

1. Uphill or stair sprints: 6 X 30" (2-3 minutes rest between each sprint)

Short 3'-5' break (set up equipment)

2. *Superset Dips and Inverted-rows (4 sets)*

   a) Dips: 4 – 15 reps

   b) Inverted-rows: 4-20 reps

3. Side to Side Hollow body rocks: 15" – 60"

<u>Workout C (Friday)</u>

A. Pull-ups: 3 sets Rest-pause sets, 4 - 30+ reps

B. Push-ups: 3 Rest-pause sets, 4 - 30+ reps

<u>Workout D (Saturday)</u>

A. Dips: 3 Rest-pause sets, 4 - 30+ reps

B. Inverted rows: 3 Rest-pause sets, 4 - 30+ reps

Done with the advanced phase – Now what?

First of all, if you went through all three phases successfully – congratulations! This means that you've trained consistently for more than six months, and as a result you've gained a lot of strength, muscle and an overall striking calisthenics physique. Right now, I highly recommend that you take a ten to fourteen-day break and allow your body to fully recover. Joints, connective tissue and your neuromuscular system deserve a break. Also, as we mentioned earlier in the book, your body needs maintenance periods and time off every now and then. Chronic high-volume training will only desensitize your muscles to muscle-growth and increase potential risk of overuse injuries.

At this point, maintaining a stable fit lifestyle is fairly easy. If you want to continue to progress, you'll have to continue to push yourself quite hard. This is a decision you should take based on what phase of your life you're in (in terms of work, school, family-responsibilities, general emotional state, etc.). You first need to think about your priorities. Is training harder and investing a lot of time in your workouts something that will add or subtract value from your life?

Maybe you feel motivated to keep on challenging yourself because you're excited with all your progress so far. Maybe you're struggling emotionally with a breakup or financial issues and pushing it hard with your training allows you to diffuse some of that negative emotional charge. If something like that is the case, then go for it!

Or... maybe your time and energy resources are limited, and balancing things a bit is a wiser option. For example, you might have a lot of other things going on and your time is limited. Maybe you have very important exams... Or maybe your wife is pregnant... Maybe you have to move to a new house. Hey, maybe you want to spare some time and energy and invest it in improving another part of your life, now that you're already in good shape. Perhaps you want to develop a new skill, such as learning to play the piano or learning a martial art? That's great as well!

To keep building muscle...
After your time off, introduce training again gradually back into your weekly schedule. Start with basic beginner volume for a week (10 sets per movement pattern). After that go through microcycle 3 of Macrocycle A from the Intermediate Phase. Next move to Macrocycle B and from there continue for the rest of the plan. You can go through the advanced phase twice a year, but not more than that. During the rest of the year stick to maintenance volume as shown below.

For Maintenance...
Your first two weeks you want to allow your body to readjust to training again. Start with basic beginner volume for a week (10 sets per movement pattern). Next, I'll offer you two maintenance workout plans. One for those who prefer training three days a week and one for those who prefer the same four-day frequency that most of this book followed.

MAINTENANCE FOUR-DAY PLAN

Workout A1 (Monday)
Circuit training (3 sets)
  a) Pull-ups: 4 – 12 reps
  b) Push-ups: 4-20 reps
  c) Plyo-Burpees: 8 – 30 reps

Workout B1 (Tuesday)
Circuit Training (3 sets)
  a) Dips: 4 – 15 reps
  b) Inverted-rows: 4-20 reps
  c) Jumping lunges: 5 – 30 reps

Workout A2 (Thursday)
1. Uphill or stair sprints: 4 X 30" (2-3 minutes rest between each sprint)
   Short 3'-5' break (set up equipment)
2. *Superset Pull-up and push-ups (3 sets)*
  a) Pull-ups: 4 – 12 reps

b) Push-ups: 4 - 20 reps
2. Hollow body side to side rocks: 15 – 60 seconds

Workout B2 (Friday)
   1. Uphill or stair sprints: 4 X 30" (2-3 minutes rest between each sprint)
     Short 3'-5' break (set up equipment)
   2. Superset Dips and Inverted-rows (3 sets)
   a) Dips: 4 – 15 reps
   b) Inverted-rows: 4 -20 reps
   2. Angel of Death: 3 sets, 8-20 reps

MAINTENANCE THREE-DAY PLAN

Workout A (Monday)
1. Uphill or stair sprints: 4 X 30" (2-3 minutes rest between each sprint)
   Short 3'-5' break (set up equipment)
2. Superset Pull-up and push-ups (3 sets)
a) Pull-ups: 4 – 12 reps
b) Push-ups: 4 - 20 reps
3. Hollow body side to side rocks: 15 – 60 seconds

Workout B (Wednesday)
Circuit training (3 sets)
a) Pull-ups: 4 – 12 reps
b) Jumping lunges: 5-30 reps
c) Push-ups: 4-20 reps
d) Plyo-Burpees: 8 – 30 reps

Workout C (Friday)
1. Uphill or stair sprints: 4 X 30" (2-3 minutes rest between each sprint)
   Short 3'-5' break (set up equipment)
2. *Superset Dips and Inverted-rows (3 sets)*
a) Dips: 4 – 15 reps
b) Inverted-rows: 4 -20 reps
3. Angel of Death: 3 sets, 8-20 reps

Exercise considerations for long-term bodyweight training
After training consistently for a year, it's a good idea to add some more rotational training to your core training. Woodchoppers are a great one. You can do these with bands, a dumbbell or even a rock if you're training outdoors.

BUILDING YOUR OWN PERSONALIZED PLAN

If the format of this plan doesn't suit your daily schedule or preferences, you can make adjustments to it. Maybe you prefer a three-day or a six-day training frequency, instead of the typical four-day frequency that is used. If you use the same training volume and follow all the basic bodyweight muscle principles we talked about in this book, there won't be a big difference in your workout's effectiveness.

Other good reasons to make adjustments to the plan are because of stress levels, age, demanding jobs (physically or even mentally), or bad genetics (i.e. maybe your recovery rates are a lot slower than average). All these can affect how much intensity and volume your body can handle. For example, one of my trainees Michael has an unusually slow neuromuscular recovery rate. He has periods that he constantly feels tired and the training volume he can handle is quite low. Although he's done tons of medical tests, his doctors haven't found anything so far. Instead of feeling disappointed and quitting, Michael and I worked around that. We constantly adjusted his workouts and focus on consistency and calibration, instead of overtraining. Although progress is a lot slower than average, over the last two years we've managed to build a respectable amount of muscle and decent levels of strength for someone of his age. Michael is 54.

Sometimes it's important to calibrate to your situation. You might have to increase or decrease the training volume and intensity to see how your body responds. Fine-tuning a program for me is an art and you need time and experience to develop it. What's most important is that your training plan fits your lifestyle and becomes part of it. For those who often ask, I no longer do online coaching, since my face-to-face personal-training practice takes a large part of my time nowadays. I do spare some time for consults through Skype though. You can learn more about that at www.bodyweightmuscle.com/contact.

Final thoughts on program design
Remember that the recommendations in this book are not set in stone. As we said, how much training volume is ideal for each person depends on multiple factors such as recovery-rate, sleep quality, mental stress levels, nutrition, genetics... these are all things that can affect performance.

If I had to summarize hypertrophy training in five simple words, it would be "Train hard and train enough!" *Hard* as in focused, high-intensity reps that bring you close to momentary muscle failure (MMF). *Enough* as in getting adequate training volume on a weekly basis. Based on all the latest research on hypertrophy, these are the two biggest muscle-growth drivers. A lot of research is still emerging on these topics. Each new study is another piece of a big puzzle that is becoming clearer and clearer the last two decades. This means that we increasingly develop a better understanding of how programming can be tweaked to maximize results. To stay posted with these developments and how they can be applied to bodyweight training – follow me on Instagram, subscribe to my YouTube channel and subscribe to my newsletter at www.bodyweight muscle.com.

In the end, there is no one size fits all perfect training system. But, this is one of the most scientifically-based and structured programs on building muscle through bodyweight exercise that you can find currently. Follow it step by step and I guarantee you results. If you want to experiment with your own program design, but you have no training/education on these topics, here's what I recommend... Study all the muscle-building principles that I shared with you in this book. After that go through the workout plan at least once. Next, feel free to start experimenting by making little tweaks. Always be cautious and put your physical health and safety above anything else.

BOOK OUTRO

Before I end this book, I want to talk about the mental aspect of bodyweight training. Those who have been following me for a while, know that Bodyweight Muscle is not just about muscle. One of the most underrated aspects of calisthenics are the mental benefits. Most of us nowadays have a lifestyle that is unnatural for our brains and bodies. We spend too much time caged indoors, sitting under fluorescent lights. Our flight or fight system is still triggered daily, but it doesn't have the change to diffuse. Instead of running or fighting we just sit – we are static. As a result, tension in our bodies builds up. Stress levels rise and they end up fueling negative thoughts and emotions.

Outdoor training – One of the best natural antidepressants
Exercise is one of the best ways to lower stress levels. It also releases natural brain chemicals that make you feel better. For example, endorphins (neurotransmitters that activate your brain's reward system and minimize pain) are your body's natural opioid. They appear to be involved in positive emotions at moderate levels and can even modulate negative emotions. Strength circuits and high intensity uphill and upstairs running are great ways to get a good dose of these chemicals. All this enhances your sense of well-being and keeps cortisol (your body's stress hormone) levels at bay. And although most forms of exercise have these benefits, bodyweight exercise has an advantage over most. Bodyweight exercise can be done anywhere, and most importantly it can be done outside. When it comes to the mental benefits of exercise, training outdoors is way more effective to training indoors. Training outdoors in natural light, fresh air, and especially if you have the luxury – in nature, is one of the best anti-depressive activities there is.

As shown in studies, people who exercise in natural environments experience greater feelings of revitalization and greater decreases in tension, confusion and anger. Especially when it comes to mood and severe cases such as depression, while any form of physical activity helps, there is growing evidence showing how physical activity in nature has larger positive effects.

Outdoor training increases motivation and energy levels. It can improve eye-health and lower blood pressure. It leads to increased creativity, focus, memory and problem-solving skills... and the list goes on. I could write a whole new chapter on outdoor training but that is not the main purpose of this book. It is a topic I am currently working for one of my future books. Till then, if you're interested into learning more about outdoor training benefits you can google "bodyweightmuscle.com outdoor training benefits" and you'll find both a video on YouTube and detailed article on my blog.

Give it time...

It's sad to see how many people miss out on all the mental benefits that exercise can provide, and how much it could improve their life. I think that one of the biggest reasons people fail at developing a fitness lifestyle, is because they can't move passed that initial discomfort that one experiences with training. What they fail to see is how this discomfort gradually decreases. The mind slowly changes the way it perceives this sensation and you even begin to crave fitness related discomfort!

In the end, many positive things relate to how we deal with discomfort. Learning to push through some uncomfortable feelings is important to moving forward in life and being happy. I see exercise as a way to learn how to take advantage of this pain-reward system. If you give exercise the time it needs and you incorporate it in your weekly routine for a while, slowly you'll start noticing the magic. As the weeks go by and you begin to see all the positive side-effects, your brain's reward system will embrace training discomfort more and more as something good. You'll notice a sense of accomplishment following your workout. You'll look forward to that post-workout feeling of peace.

Especially if you train early in the day, you'll see how this builds momentum for accomplishing more of your goals during the rest of the day. You'll also start appreciating and enjoying more simple daily things such as resting and eating. Your sleep will improve, and you'll start being more discerning about the kind of food you choose to fuel your body with.

Exercise also gives you a better perspective and a more positive outlook on life. By diffusing the build-up of emotions that blur your thinking, and often make things seem a lot worse than they really are, you'll be able to think clearer and make better decisions. You'll even observe less friction in your interactions with people around you.

All these are just some of the benefits. Not everyone experiences all of them, but everyone definitely has positive things to gain from exercise.

In the end, we all have our own obstacles to overcome... Either that's a missing leg, fighting with self-image problems, dealing with shadows from the past, relationships or financial issues... How much we struggle is not a matter of how great our problems compared to others. It's simply a matter of being human and having emotions. Life can be tough for everyone. Exercise is a tool though that is available to everyone. Increasing our physical fitness and gaining control over our body can help us develop confidence and a sense of self-mastery. This empowers us to further take control of our life and make more positive changes day by day.

PS: GOT QUESTIONS?

I've done my best to cover everything related to building muscle with calisthenics in this book. Still, this is the first edition of the book... That means that there are probably a few details that I have missed out. Feel free to email me at info@bodyweightmuscle.com with any of your questions related to the book, and I'll do my best to get back to you within 48 hours. That way you get your questions covered, and I can also create an FAQ for my future readers. It's a win-win!

By Anthony Arvanitakis